Mystery of the Bones:

SYPHILIS, THE LEWIS AND CLARK EXPEDITION, AND THE ARIKARA INDIANS

P. WILLEY AND THOMAS P. LOWRY

Vallombrosa Press • Chico

Mystery of the Bones: Syphilis, the Lewis and Clark
Expedition, and the Arikara Indians

Vallombrosa Press, 2008
Chico, California

ISBN: 978-0-6151-9033-4

Design and production by Judy Stolen

*Cover Illustration: George Catlin "Kah-beck-a, The Twin,
Wife of Bloody Hand" 1832*

Dedication

A book is the product not only of the authors and their literary and scientific forebears, but also of a largely unseen network of supporters and encouragers, in our case, wives.

Judy Stolen's patience with this and other projects, her skills with sometimes inscrutable computers, her flair with graphic arts, and her enduring affection and charm, all form an essential background for this work.

Beverly Ann Lowry's years of devoted work in the National Archives, her skills in researching arcana, her talents in creating databases, and her affectionate and comforting presence over several decades, form the foundation for this and many other historical writings.

To them we owe a loving and enduring debt.

PW

TPL

Contents

Table of Contents v
List of Illustrations vii
List of Tables ix
Preface xi
Acknowledgments xiii
1. Introduction 1
2. Other Early Observers 9
3. Reasons for Sexual Availability 20
    Hospitality and Generosity 20
    Prostitution 22
        Sex Middlemen 24
        Prostitutes 30
        Beads 33
        Clients 35
    Transmit Spiritual Power 38
    Arikara Sex 42
    Summary 47
4. The Wages of Licentious Sex 48
    Accounts of Venereal Disease from the Lewis and Clark
      Expedition 51
    Other Accounts of Venereal Disease among Arikara 54
    Clinical Expression of Venereal Diseases 59
    Skeletal Expressions of Venereal Syphilis and Gonorrhea 63
    Summary 68
5. The Bones That Didn't Speak 70
    Arikara Villages and Lodges 71
    Arikara and the Aboriginal Trade Network 74
    Leavenworth Site and Its Skeletons 78
    Syphilis on the Plains? 84

6. Historic and Ethnographic Explanations 88
    Erroneous Historic Diagnoses 89
    Ready Remedies 92
        Doctors 92
        Illness 95
        Cures 95
    Different Mortuary Treatment for Afflicted 107
    Summary 114
7. Skeletal and Biological Explanations 115
    Erroneous Osteological Conclusions 116
    Constitutional Resistance to Disease 119
        Population Decline in Native Americans 119
        Smallpox 121
        Origin of Syphilis 123
        Syphilis and ABO Blood Types 125
    Arikara Too Short-Lived for Advanced Stages of Syphilis 129
        Life Expectancy 130
        Syphilis in the Bone 132
        Syphilis Rates 133
    Limitations of Skeleton 134
        Problems with Skeletal Age Estimations 134
        Problems Identifying Disease in the Skeleton 136
        Leavenworth Site Skeletons and Syphilis 138
    Change in Syphilitic Manifestations 140
    Summary 142
8. Discussion 143
    PreColumbian or Columbian Origin of Syphilis? 144
    Native American Graves and Repatriation Act 145
    Venereal Disease Other than Syphilis 149
    Summary 150
9. Summary and Conclusions 151
    Historic Accounts 152
    Arikara Skeletons 154
    Historic and Ethnographic Explanations 155
    Skeletal and Biological Explanations 157
    Conclusions 158
References Cited 161
Index 171

List of Illustrations

1. Map of Great Plains showing tribal territories. 2

2. Map of the Dakotas showing Leavenworth Site and other important locations. 3

3. John Bradbury. 13

4. Edward Curtis's "Arikara Maiden." 31

5. Edward Curtis's "On the Banks of the Missouri." 39

6. Daytime Smoker, a Nez Perce who claimed to be the son of William Clark. 49

7. Timeline relating Lewis and Clark Expedition's Arikara visit and appearance of VD. 50

8. F.V. Hayden, physician, who visited the Upper Missouri River Region in the mid-1800s. 57

9. Mid-19th century lithograph of syphilitic male victim showing secondary stages of disease. 61

10. Mid-19th century lithograph of syphilitic female victim showing idiosyncratic disease manifestations. 62

11. Skull vault showing caries sicca caused by tertiary syphilis. 65

12. Facial skeleton destruction from growth alterations associated with congenital syphilis. 66

13. Tibia showing bowing ("saber shin") associated with tertiary syphilis. 67

14. Catlin's drawing of the bank villages where Lewis and Clark visited the Arikara and where skeletons were excavated. 72

15. Maurice Kirby's map of the Leavenworth Site. 80

16. University of Kansas archaeologists of the Leavenworth Site, summer 1965. 82

17. Edward Curtis's "In the Medicine-lodge." 93

18. Edward Curtis's "Contents of Arikara Tribal Medicine Bundle." 96

19. Melvin R. Gilmore, University of Michigan ethnobotoanist. 100

20. Purple coneflower (*Echinacea angustifolia*). 106

21. Arikara population decline from the mid-18th century through the early 20th century. 121

List of Tables

Table 1. Skeletal remains excavated from Leavenworth Site. 79

Table 2. Plants used by Native Americans to treat venereal diseases. 98-99

Table 3. Bradbury's list of plant materials identified in Arikara medicine man's bundle, June 14, 1811. 103

Table 4. ABO blood type frequencies in 20th century Full Blood Pawnee and Caddo living in Oklahoma. 129

Table 5. Expected number of Leavenworth Site skeletons having syphilitic lesions. 139

Preface

The Bones That Wouldn't Speak

The spade confirms the myth. That is the traditional marriage of legend and archaeology.

For centuries–actually millennia–Troy was thought to be the mere creation of a blind poet, who himself may not have existed. But, in 1870 Heinrich Schliemann put his spade into the soil of western Turkey and found not only one but many Troys. Just six years later, he unearthed the gold of the Mycenaeans who ruled Bronze Age Greece 3500 years ago. The Homeric era was real.

In Egypt, Imhotep had long been worshiped as a god of healing and architecture, a far cry from his cinematic role in "Return of the Mummy." The real mythical Imhotep was architect to Pharaoh Djoser, who was buried in the famous pyramid at Sakkara. Or so the legend went, until Imhotep's name was found in Djoser's tomb. Imhotep was real, not a myth.

Careful excavation of the bones and cartridges at the Little Bighorn site has confirmed some battle stories and disproved others, in the endless search for the real story of Custer's last stand. The excavation of mass graves has confirmed stories of the Black Death in England and of Saddam's atrocities in Iraq.

Excavations at Traveler's Rest, a spot where the Lewis and Clark Expedition camped and recuperated, have found a pit with a high level of mercury. The surrounding soils have no mercury. The pit is almost certainly the expedition's latrine and the mercury almost certainly from the pills administered to the men to treat syphilis.

Earlier in the expedition, Lewis and Clark had stopped for the winter at the Mandan villages. Within days of arriving among the Mandans, the journals report an outbreak of syphilis, a disease whose usual incubation period is three weeks. The expedition had been in the Arikara villages just three weeks before arriving among the Mandans. A reasonable conclusion is that this episode of syphilis reflected disease caught among the Arikaras.

Many studies have shown that syphilis alters many anatomical structures, including the bones. Therefore, the bones of early 19th century Arikara Indians should also bear these syphilitic stigmata. But they do not!

How can this be? Why does the evidence of the spade–the carefully studied bones–not confirm the clearly recorded observations of the two famous captains, both meticulous diarists? The attempt to unravel this mystery will lead us to several subsidiary and equally vital questions:

- Medical understanding of venereal disease in 1804.
- Evidence of venereal disease among the Arikaras.
- Evidence that the Arikaras were willing to share their sexual favors (and illnesses) with visitors.
- Evidence for the absence of venereal disease in the Lewis and Clark Expedition before arriving at the Arikara villages.
- Possible errors in the Lewis and Clark journals.
- The current science of paleopathology, or how to read the bones.
- Limitations in the science of identifying disease in bones.

A careful consideration of all these questions may enable us to answer The Mystery of the Bones.

Acknowledgments

J ack T. Hughes (1921-2001), the "Dean" of Panhandle archaeology who spent his career at West Texas State, once said that including people in acknowledgments was an inexpensive way of thanking those folks who provided invaluable help. Acknowledgments, as he claimed, are inexpensive, but we believe they are a no-less heart-felt means of recognizing essential assistance. We are much indebted to the individuals mentioned below as well as many others too numerous to list.

We thank Miss Roberts, social studies teacher for many years at Central Junior High School, Lawrence, Kansas. More than 45 years ago, following seventh grader P's extemporaneous in-class discussion, she took him aside in the school hallways to explain that the disease which Columbus may or may not have possessed did not begin with the letter C and that disease had a more complicated mode of transmission than the youth could have imagined. She was right on both counts.

William M. Bass's University of Kansas's archaeological excavations at the Arikara Leavenworth Site cemeteries in 1965 and 1966 were seminal times for Great Plains bioarchaeology. Changes were afoot that we hardly could have imagined and the questions we were asking then have led to many even more intriguing puzzles, one of which we address in this book.

Douglas H. Ubelaker, Smithsonian Institution, corresponded with us and clarified our interpretations concerning his descriptions of Leavenworth Site dental remains. Richard L. Jantz, University of Tennessee-Knoxville (UT-K), provided suggestions concerning Arikara ABO blood types. Lee Meadows Jantz, UT-K, provided notes from historic accounts that P wrote in 1975 and 1976 while he was employed at UT-K.

Jim Bauml of the Los Angeles Arboretum provided detailed information on medicinal plants of the Great Plains, and David Wood and Kristina Schierenbeck of Chico State's Biological Sciences Department also aided our botanical efforts.

Jeff Thomas, physician at Chico State's Student Health Services, discussed present-day venereal diseases and their treatment in a young adult population. Charlie Urbanowicz, Chico State's Anthropology Department, provided information and leads on Melanesian cargo cults.

Jim Merril, former editor of *We Proceeded On*, was instrumental in this work. Had he accepted our proposal for a manuscript in June 2006, rather than postponing the decision for his successor, we probably would not have bothered writing this lengthy volume. We also thank Wendy Raney, the current editor of that journal, for publishing a much abbreviated version of this book under the article "The Mystery of the Bones" (*We Proceeded On* 33:22-26, January 2007).

Our work on syphilis and the Arikara bones has been orally presented. We gave talks at Chico State ("Lewis and Clark, VD, and the Arikara Bones," Anthropology 497 Anthropology Forum, September 21, 2006; and "Syphilis in the Arikara Bones," Anthropology 600

Core Seminar in Anthropology, September 25, 2006 and September 11, 2007). We also presented a paper at the Plains Anthropological Conference ("Lewis and Clark Expedition, Syphilis, and Arikara Osteology," Topeka, KS, November 2006). Chico State's College of Behavioral and Social Sciences' Professional Development Committee provided partial funding to cover expenses associated with attending the Plains Anthropological Conference. We are grateful to the attendees of those presentations and those who had kind questions and made valuable suggestions, especially Linea Sundstrom. Their interest and ideas helped clarify our thoughts and directions.

1. Introduction

As the Lewis and Clark Expedition traveled up the Missouri River, their journals reflected encounters with three different tribes (Fig. 1). In early August 1804, they met the Otoes, but recorded no carnal transactions. In late September, their Teton Dakota hosts at least twice offered the captains young women as bed partners. The Dakota were puzzled—even offended—when the captains spurned the invitations. Did other men of the expedition receive such an offer? And if they did, were the invitations accepted? Here, the journals are silent.

In mid-October, the expedition spent time with the Arikara at their villages (Figs. 1 and 2), where sexual activity occurred. Both Sgt. Patrick Gass and Capt. Clark recorded the Arikara custom of welcoming travelers by providing women, and noted specifically that, "the men by means of interpreters found no difficulty in getting women." Lewis added, "Their women verry fond of caressing our men etc." York, Clark's African-American slave, was perceived by the Arikaras as possessing "magic," and at least one Arikara husband arranged to have his wife receive York's mystical powers.

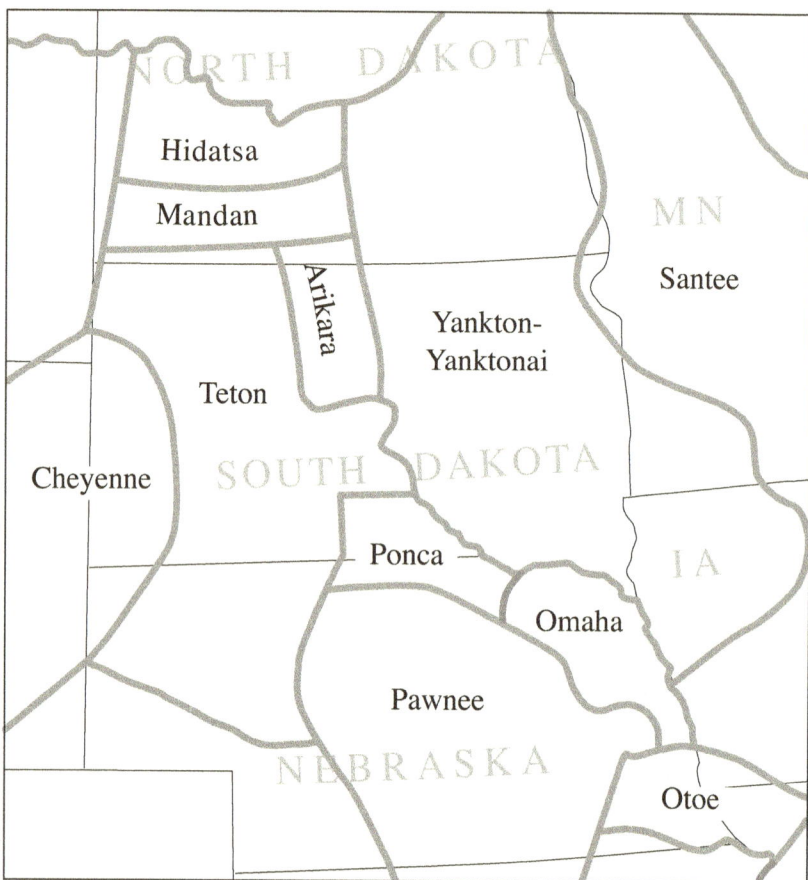

Figure 1. Map of Great Plains showing tribal territories. (Modified from DeMallie 2001:ix).

Similar encounters were recorded when the expedition wintered with the Mandan.

The expedition's Arikara sojourn occurred with an indigenous group whose pastime and livelihood was entertaining and trading with many peoples from a variety of cultural backgrounds, most of whom were trail weary, having traveled long distances (Ewers 1968, Ronda 1984:42-66). The Arikara were the consummate traders, making a K-Mart blue-light special seem lackluster by contrast. And they were just as hospitable, leaving many visitors empty-pocketed

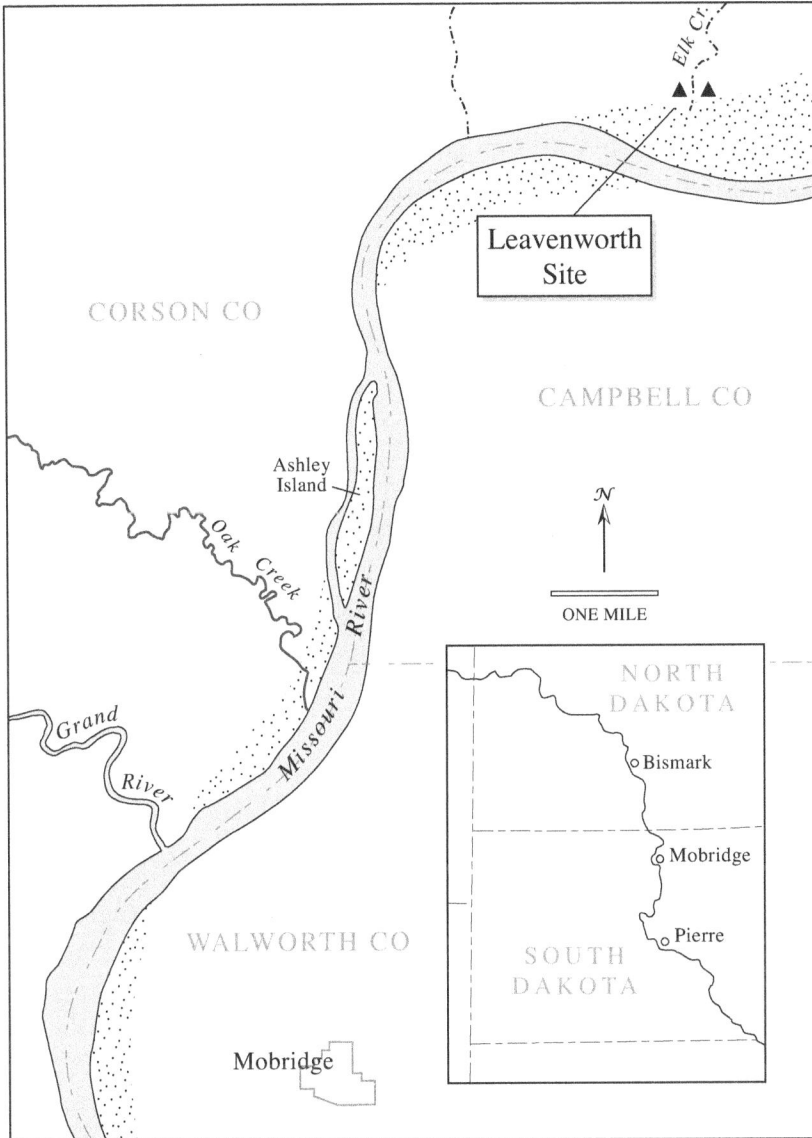

Figure 2. Map of the Dakotas showing Leavenworth Site and other important locations. (After Wedel 1955:76, fig. 10).

and grinning as they departed the Arikara villages. The Arikara, in short, put Southern hospitality to shame.

The Arikara villages were one of two major indigenous trading centers on the Upper Missouri River, the other being the Mandan-

Hidatsa villages farther upriver in present-day North Dakota. From the south and west, tribes came to the Arikara, among them the Cheyenne as noted by Lewis and Clark (Moulton 2002, 3:403). These southerly and western groups ultimately had contact with the Spanish settlements in the Southwest and through the Spanish they had access to horses—the key posession of the Plains equestrian nomads.

From the west and south, the Arikaras' major trading partners were Teton Dakota and through them the other Dakota groups further to the east. Those groups had access to guns, another critical item in the historic period. In addition to the horse and gun, the Arikara trade included many indigenous goods, such as meat, flour, and painted robes (Ewers 1968). It is likely that the trade of these indigenous items stretched far into the prehistoric past (Blakeslee 1981), with the Euroamerican trade goods only the most recent veneer on that long list of swapped items, comparable to the shiny new things in a flea market.

One aspect of trade, a mechanism that lubricated the wheels of commerce, was Arikara hospitality. Many travelers recorded the Arikaras' generosity, especially noting they provided the arriving visitors, their guests, with food, gifts and lodging.

Among many traditional groups, generosity and giving were emphasized, even to the detriment of accumulation of material goods. A wealthy person from their perspective might acquire desirable goods, but their importance was in being given away, not in the accumulation itself. The Arikara, for one, emphasized generosity and giving, avoiding the accumulation of material wealth for its own sake. We have difficulty comprehending such generosity just as the Arikara had a hard time understanding why anyone might think otherwise.

Comments recorded by Pierre Antoine Tabeau (Abel 1939:134-135), a trader who was living in the Arikara villages during the Lewis and Clark Expedition's Arikara respite in October 1804, are telling along these lines. He wrote, their "minds, not grasping our ideas of interest and acquisition beyond what is necessary, it is a principle with them that he who has divides with him who has not." Such notions of generosity must have frustrated many a Euroamerican trader, whose free-market goal was to accumulate as many furs and hides as possible, and to maximize profits. A related frustration affected the white traders' Arikara hosts.

Tabeau (1939:135) provided an Arikara perspective on the trade, relayed to him by an Arikara.

> "You are foolish," said one of the most intelligent seriously to me. "Why do you wish to make all this powder and these balls since you do not hunt? Of what use are all these knives to you? Is it not enough with which to cut the meat? It is only your wicked heart that prevents you from giving them to us. Do you not see that the village has none? I will give you a robe myself, when you want it, but you already have more robes than are necessary to cover you."

A wealthy and socially responsible Arikara man was one who provided for the less fortunate, whether the impoverished person needed food, knives or buffalo robes—even to the point of impoverishing himself.

One aspect of this hospitality and generosity was the Arikara womens' sexual availability. Gass and Clark noted this behavior during the expedition's October 1804 lay over with the Arikara.

On October 12, 1804, Sgt. Patrick Gass (Lowry 2004:58), who kept a journal and published it in 1807, after commenting the previous day about the Arikara women's beauty, noted that the Arikara had an "unusual custom of showing appreciation." Clark provided more details about this unusual custom.

On October 12, 1804, the same day as Gass's note, Clark (Moulton 2003: 57) wrote

> a curious Cuistom with the Souix [Dakota] as well as the reckeres [Arikara] is to give handsom Squars to those whome they wish to Show Some acknowledgements to—The Seauix we got Clare of without taking their Squars, they followed us with Squars . . . two days. The Rickores we put off duering the time we were at the Towns but 2 Handsom young Squars were Sent by a man to follow us, they Came up this evening and persisted in their Civilities.

Although Clark implied that there was no sexual contact between the expedition members and the Arikaras—at least not in the villages and at least not as a gift—he seemed to suggest that there may have been such congress either not as a gift or as they continued their journey upriver from the villages.

Contrasted with Clark's previous comments, Biddle's version of the Arikara visit is more explicit concerning these relations. There Clark (Biddle 1814:105) wrote "These women are handsomer than the Sioux; both are however, disposed to be amourous, and our men found no difficulty in procuring companions for the night by means of the interpreters. These interviews were chiefly clandestined, and were of course to be kept secret from the husbands or relations." Presumably these "interviews" occurred in the Arikara villages and before the previously mentioned in-transit propositions occurred while proceeding up the river.

Clark probably refers to the same incident in another context. As the expedition departed the Arikara villages in October 1804, Clark noted that "2 young Squars verry anxious to accompany us" (Moulton 2002, 3:175). The reason for attempting to hitch a ride up the Missouri is unclear; one reason would be to initiate or continue sexual relations, another reason to get a free ride upriver. It is further unclear whether the two young women actually did accompany the expedition or just expressed their desire to do so. But whether or not these women accompanied the expedition, there were sexually transmitted microbes that did accompany some expedition members, getting a free ride up the Missouri River, as they traveled up some of the men's urogenital tracts.

A few days later, the expedition arrived at a small Arikara camp upriver from the main Arikara villages. There Clark (Moulton 2003: 59) noted "Their womin verry fond of caressing our men," perhaps a reference to being attracted to Clark's black servant, York, and other expedition men.

York may have had the best time at the Arikara villages of any of the expedition's men—perhaps the best time he had on the entire trip. He was apparently the first black person the Arikara had seen, and as such was a mystery or "medicine" to them. He played to the Arikara preconceptions, telling them that he had been a wild animal until Clark captured and tamed him. Before that, York claimed, he had subsisted on people, children making the best eating of all (Moulton 2003:55). York's "magic" was too much for the Arikara to resist, one husband arranging for York to have sex with his wife while the man stood guard to prevent anyone from interrupting (Jackson 1978, 2: 503).

Such offers may have seemed odd, as well as flattering, to the captains and the men. But they were transient visitors among the Arikara, there for only a brief period, and relied on interpreters both for linguistic translations as well as cultural explanations. So, did Lewis and Clark get it right? Were the Arikara, as their accounts claim, sexually licentious? And among the consequences of such sexual availability were there venereal diseases that the journals mention?

Expedition members mentioned sexually transmitted diseases that may have been contracted from the Arikara. Venereal disease symptoms were noted the month after visiting the Arikara and again two months later. What was the disease or diseases they experienced?

We use a variety of sources to assess these questions. The accounts of other early travelers, trappers, and traders provide support for many of the expedition's observations as well as other reasons and additional details, especially those concerning Arikara culture and behavior. Some other historic accounts also include descriptions of venereal diseases, the inevitable consequence of such sexual license. In addition to the other historic accounts, there are other approaches to assessing the expedition members' descriptions.

Archaeology and osteology provide material evidence, not so susceptible to distortion, as cultural, linguistic and written interpretations. The material evidence of artifacts and bones is used to assess the written documents, although, as the reader will see, the bones prove ambiguous themselves. And they indicate that venereal diseases were not present in the early 19th century Arikara. But first, before we delve into the tangible bones, what can we learn from the other visitors' accounts of the Arikara in addition to those of the members of the Lewis and Clark Expedition?

2. Other Early Observers

L ewis and Clark were not the first whites to meet the Arikara. And neither were they the first travelers to note the hospitality of the Arikara and the sexual availability of their women. Traders and other travelers of the period made similar observations.

Some of the traders spent time with the Arikara, living in their villages, exchanging manufactured goods for furs, eating their food, and sharing their beds. These white men had dealings and first-hand experience with the Arikara that often lasted months. During their stays, they bartered and bargained with the Arikara, a swap that included materials as well as services such as sex.

Travelers, on the other hand, were usually just passing through Arikara country as part of longer voyages. In some cases, their experiences with the Arikara, as those of Lewis and Clark, were little better than the 19th century version of a 21st century tourist who has been there, done that, sent the postcards, and bought the tee shirt. Not that they were above swapping materials and sex with the Arikara— they were not. It is just that travelers' exposure to the let's-make-a-deal atmosphere of the Arikara villages was of shorter duration and more comparable to the expedition's experience than that of traders. Travelers were, after all, on tour and had miles to go before reaching the next photo opportunity.

Much of what we know about the early 19th century Arikara comes from these traders' and travelers' observations and the written records they left. It behooves us to introduce these diarists, presenting them in the chronological sequence they met the Arikara. In addition to introducing the observers, portions of their accounts concerning sex and the Arikara are presented here; their additional observations concerning Arikara sexual practices and their consequences are considered in later chapters.

Although having been in direct contact with EuroAmericans since the 1730s, the earliest detailed account concerning the Arikara was left by Jean Baptiste Trudeau (1914:460-461). He was a trader from St. Louis, who spent time with the Arikara during the summer of 1795, the decade before the Lewis and Clark Expedition poled up the Missouri River.

Born on December 11, 1748, in Montreal, Trudeau was middle aged that summer. As a young man, he moved from Canada to St. Louis, where he established and managed a boys' school that continued for approximately 45 years. His school, located in his home—the Trudeau House, was on the grounds where the St. Louis Gateway Arch now stands. His house and school were gateways to the Arikara and other Missouri River Indians as well as the West, and the foundation he built remains a gateway today.

Despite being occupied as school master in St. Louis, Trudeau claimed more than 25 years' experience trading with tribes on the Missouri River and its tributaries. The impetus for his Arikara trip began when the Company of Explorers was formed in May 1794; the following month Trudeau and eight men castoff from St. Louis, planning to trade with the Arikara and other tribes above the Ponca (Fig. 1).

Traveling upriver, belligerent Teton Dakota forced them ashore in late September 1794. The Teton held them for several days and extorted goods before the traders were allowed to pass. After a failed attempt to reach the Arikara upriver, Trudeau and his party drifted down the Missouri River, to a place below the Teton and above the Omaha where they wintered (1794-95). In early spring 1795 the party left their winter quarters and traveled to the Arikara villages, located near the mouth of the Grand River. The Arikara had recently been forced upriver to that location from their villages in central South Dakota by fighting with the Dakota and the devastating effects of epidemic diseases. Trudeau and company settled with the Arikara while they awaited arrival of boats from St. Louis. Presumably the boats arrived, although his journal omits their arrival and it abruptly ends. From what can be inferred from other sources, the party pushed further upriver and spent the next winter (1795-96) with Mandan. Then they drifted downstream to the place where they spent the first winter between the Teton and Omaha and stayed there during the subsequent winter (1796-97).

By 1798 Trudeau was back to his school and his teaching duties in St. Louis. Lewis and Clark presumably consulted with Trudeau during the winter of 1803-04, which they spent near St. Louis, and they probably carried a copy of his journal with them on their journey. Trudeau's perspective on the Arikara was an early and engaged one. Further, Trudeau may have influenced Lewis and Clark's views of the Arikara, even before the expedition rowed beyond the outskirts of St. Louis.

Trudeau, as others, noted Arikara sexual behavior. He (1914: 460-461) wrote

The girls and young women who seem to be common property among them, living in full liberty, are so dissolute and debauched that, according to the reports of those who have studied them, there is not one whose modesty is proof against a bit of vermillion or a few strands of blue glass beads; what is more, the fathers, brothers and even the husbands offer and take the youngest and most beautiful daughters, sisters and wives to the white Men for their diversion, in exchange for a few trifles which they receive.

In another place, Trudeau indicated that such commerce was not new, but stretched back at least a few years (Trudeau 1914:457). So, Trudeau noted the Arikara's sexual availability, especially to whites, as part of a trade relationship—themes we will return to in future chapters.

Pierre Antoine Tabeau was a later trader with the Arikara (Abel 1939:180-181). He was living with the Arikara in an island village when Lewis and Clark visited. His presence there was acknowledged by Clark, mentioning him as "Mr Taboe" (October 9, 1804; Moulton 2003:54) and "Mr. Tabo" (October 10, 1804; Moulton 2003:55). He left the Arikara villages most likely in 1805 and was in St. Louis by September 1806 to welcome the returning expedition members at the conclusion of their journey to the Pacific Ocean.

Tabeau was born January 15, 1755 in Lachine, Montreal, and attended a seminary in Quebec. He, however, was destined to be a trader of goods, not a saver of souls—a salvation for his potential parishioners considering his acerbic personality. While in his early 20s, he became an engagé and a few years later he was working with his brother as a trader. When he lived with the Arikara, he was employed by Loisel's company of St. Louis. James Mackay (in Abel 1939:11) described Tabeau as "an infamous rascal" for misdeeds, and his acerbic writings lend support to this label. Tabeau had a perspective

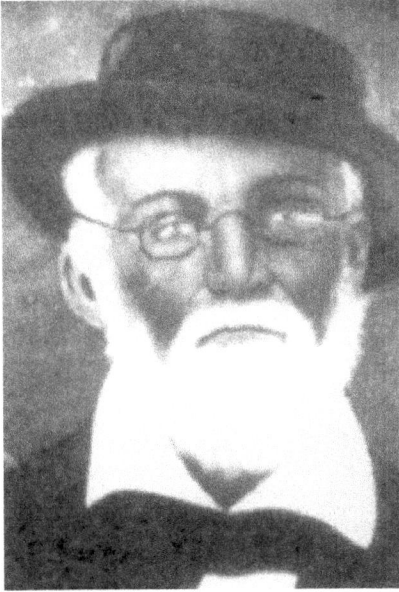

Figure 3. John Bradbury, the botanist who visited the Arkara in 1811 and made observations concerning medicinal uses of plants.

of the Arikara that only a resident—and perhaps only an infamous rascal—could.

Tabeau (Abel 1939:180-181) confirmed the availability of Arikara women. He wrote "This politeness [sexual activity] is carried out every day among the Ricaras, and always the more readily in the case of the whites;.... [It] is said that the girls are virtuous before marriage and that there are virgins, eighteen to twenty years old. Truth exceeds probability here." If Tabeau was correct, then there were few, if any, chaste Arikara women. And unless the sexual traffic was limited to Arikara women and their white men consorts (those Caucasoid gods!), similar sexual activity probably occurred with the Arikara men as well as many of the other male visitors to the Arikara villages. They were undoubtedly sexually active too.

In addition to the two just-mentioned traders, travelers also visited the Arikara and noted their behavior. John Bradbury (Fig. 3) visited the Arikara in the decade after Tabeau's stay and

Lewis and Clark's visit. (http://www.tameside.gov.uk/leisure/newbp_05.htmm).

Bradbury was a Scot born in 1768 who was largely self-schooled and made a living in the cotton industry. In his spare time he published botany articles and eventually gained such prestige that Liverpool's Philosophical Society/Botanical Society funded his journey to the United States to collect plants from 1809 to 1812.

Arriving in the US, one of his first stops was to visit Thomas Jefferson, who had just completed his second term as president. Following a 10-day stay at Monticello, Bradbury carried a letter of introduction from Jefferson to Lewis, who was then governor of the Louisiana Territory, headquartered in St. Louis. Bradbury spent the spring and summer of 1810 in the vicinity of St. Louis, collecting plants and keeping a detailed journal. In 1811 he was invited to accompany the Astorian Expedition up the Missouri River. He journeyed from St. Louis the 1800 miles to the Arikara villages, then an additional 200 miles to the Mandan before descending the Missouri River in one of Manuel Lisa's boats. His adventure of a lifetime, however, was just beginning.

After returning to St. Louis, he fell ill for four months, and in December 1811, he was traveling down the Mississippi River from St. Louis to New Orleans when the first New Madrid Earthquake struck. The New Madrid Earthquakes, beginning that year and continuing into the next year, centered near New Madrid, Missouri, and adjacent portions of Kentucky, Tennessee and Arkansas. The shocks, some of them estimated to be 8.0 magnitude on the not-then-developed Richter scale, devastated the region, with some areas sinking, and portions of the Mississippi River changing course—perhaps even running backwards for a short period. The shocks were felt over the contiguous US, excepting the West Coast, and even rang church bells

1,000 miles away in Boston. The New Madrid Earthquakes were much stronger than the 1906 San Francisco Earthquake.

As if natural disasters including fever and one of the most severe earthquake in contiguous-US history were not enough, while he was preparing to leave the US and return to England, international political events intervened. War between the US and England erupted, preventing his departure. His plant collection preceded him, however, and arrived safely in England. When he finally did return home, he discovered that many of his plants had already been described and published by an unscrupulous botanist, Frederick Pursh. Despite this disappointment, he busied himself writing *Travels in the Interior of America in the Years 1809, 1810, and 1811*, which was published in 1817. It sold poorly, impoverishing him and his family. Professionally and financially broken, he returned to the US and St. Louis, perhaps in part to avoid his Liverpool sponsors and creditors. He did not initiate any further botanical studies, died and was initially buried in the US. Eventually his remains were disinterred and returned to England for burial (Rickett 1950, Bradbury 1904).

During his first trip in the US, in addition to his collecting and other botanical duties, Bradbury noted other aspects of American natural history and social behavior, including the Arikara sex trade. Concerning sexual availability, he wrote (1904:140) "In this species of liberality no nation can exceed the Arikaras, who flocked down every evening with their wives, sisters, and daughters, anxious to meet with a market for them." So Bradbury confirms what Trudeau, Lewis and Clark, and Tabeau had observed: the Arikara women were sexually available and actively involved with white men.

On the other hand, there were two counter claims to this depiction of Arikara having a sexually wide-open society and all Arikaras being debauched. Those accounts were written by other observers.

Henry Marie Brackenridge visited the Arikara villages at the same time as botanist Bradbury, the decade after Lewis and Clark, and Tabeau. Brackenridge (1906) was born in Pittsburgh in 1786, and following many far-flung travels, he died near his birthplace in 1871. As a youth, encouraged by his father, he read law, eventually practicing in Baltimore and Pennsylvania before moving to St. Louis. In 1811 he accompanied Manuel Lisa's trading company up the Missouri River to the Arikara villages, returning to St. Louis that same summer accompanying Bradbury. We will return to his visit with the Arikara momentarily after following his subsequent journeys. By 1819 his wanderings had taken him far from the Arikara, but with the purchase of Florida, he threw his lot with that territory. By 1832, however, he was back in Pittsburgh, where he spent the rest of his life.

While generally confirming their sexual availability, Brackenridge made observations indicating not all Arikara women were licentious and debauched. Brackenridge described a public rite at the villages when any Arikara woman who had "preserved unsullied her virgin purity" could claim prizes of beads, vermillion and cloth. There were some chaste women who stepped forward and walked away with the prizes (Brackenridge 1906:130-132). So, if Brackenridge was correct, there were at least some Arikara women who were not the dissolute vixens that other travelers describe.

In addition to Brackenridge, there is another counter claim. A few years after Brackenridge's visit, John C. Luttig kept a journal while chief aide and clerk at a post near the Arikara villages, Fort Manuel Lisa. Luttig is believed to be of German origin and education based on the spelling and calligraphy of his journal, although apparently little else is known about his early life (Drumm 1920: 12-14). History first finds him as a Baltimore merchant, and he was in St. Louis by 1809. He was engaged by various employers, including Governor Clark, in various positions. He changed jobs frequently, which may have been due in part to his fondness of alcohol. He died July 19, 1815, while in Lawrence, Missouri Territory, now a part of Arkansas.

Fort Manuel Lisa was established late summer 1812 a few miles above the Arikara villages and was occupied until early 1813, a period when the War of 1812 was raging. The fort was abandoned, perhaps fearing a British invasion descending from Canada down the Missouri River, to attack St. Louis and New Orleans. Their fear was well founded considering the strategic importance of the Mississippi River indicated by the 1815 Battle of New Orleans. At the very least, British were believed to be agitating Native Americans on the Upper Missouri River, encouraging them to take up arms against US traders and trappers. One event near Ft. Manuel was attributed to such agitation and may have precipitated abandonment of the fort.

In February 1813, Louis Archambeau, while hauling hay across the river from Fort Manuel Lisa, was attacked by hundreds of Sioux (Luttig 1964:125). They

> took the Scalp and cut him nearly to pieces, they marched off about 4 oclock, leaving us to lament the Death of a fellow Citizen unrevenged, a party of our Men went across to bring the Corps [sic.] which they found terrible mangled, they brought 29 Arrows which were sticking in his body and a good many more had been brocken [sic.] to pieces, his Head Broken[,] the Brains scattered about[.] his nose and ears cut off, his teeth Knocked out, and more terrible Deeds which I will not express with my Pen.

Those "more terrible deeds" may have included decapitation, dismemberment and castration. Luttig's journal itself is "decapitated," ending abruptly the following month, apparently as the company abandoned the fort and fled downriver to St. Louis.

For all of its keen observations and wealth of information, Luttig's journal is best known for possibly documenting the death of Sacagawea. She was the Shoshone woman, one of Charbonneau's wives, who was instrumental in the expedition's successful journey.

She served as guide, mediator and translator, and she and her infant's presence with the expedition was a tangible indication of the group's peaceful intentions.

Luttig's (1964:106) entry for December 20, 1812 noted "this evening the wife of Charbonneau, a Snake Squaw, died of a putrid fever[.] she was a good and the best woman in the fort, aged about 25 years. She left a fine infant girl." If the death recorded was another woman other than Sacagawea, then an alternate story goes, that Sacagawea lived a long life, dying decades later among her Shoshone people.

There is some uncertainty whether this woman was Sacagawea or one of Charbonneau's other wives. In either case, the infant was Lizette, who Luttig took to St. Louis, where Clark adopted her. Luttig died several years later in 1815.

While at Ft. Manuel Lisa, Luttig noted Arikara sexual availability, but with some qualifications. His entry two months before Charbonneau's wife died, for October 14, 1812 (Luttig 1964:85-86) reads "...some Rees arrived to trade a little Corn and a Girl[.] the first was traded but not the last, she wanted to be the Wife of Frenchman, and not his concubine,—Chastity." As Brackenridge's account of the Arikara rite previously noted, Luttig documented at least one Arikara woman who was reserved and interested in relations in the context of marriage, eschewing the sexual license others apparently embraced.

To summarize these trader and traveler tales, the accounts indicate that at least under certain circumstances some Arikara women were sexually active and available to whites. Not to over-state their availability, other women—or perhaps the same women in different social contexts— were apparently unavailable. There were several motivations for the sexual availability of Arikara women. They included hospitality, prostitution, and power transmission—topics we present in the next chapter.

3. Reasons for Sexual Availability

There are several reasons why the Arikara women were sexually available—in addition to the normal biological functions, that is. They include hospitality, prostitution, and power transmission. In this chapter we also present what little is known about sex within traditional Arikara society.

Hospitality and Generosity

As mentioned in a previous chapter, the Arikara were the hosts who knew much about hospitality—the hosts with the most, it might be said. Generosity included feeding and lodging their guests, as well as entertaining them. And entertainment sometimes included sex.

Trudeau (in Smith 1936:567), who lived with the Arikara during the decade before Lewis and Clark's visit, noted such hospitality. Husbands "fathers and brothers, are importunate with the white men who visit them, to make free with their wives, daughters and sisters, particularly those who are most youthful and pretty;…. Indeed both the girls and the married women are so loose in their conduct, that they seem to be a sort of common stock,...." And Trudeau's assessment was echoed by a later visitor to the Arikara.

Brackenridge (1906:129-130), the attorney traveler who visited the Arikara in 1811, noted "...I observed that it was a part of their hospitality, to offer the guest, who takes up his residence in their lodges, one of the females of the family as a bedfellow; sometimes even one of their wives, daughters, or sisters, but most usually a maid-servant, according to the estimation in which the guest is held, and to decline such offer is considered as treating the host with some disrespect;...." Brackenridge noted that such offers were made to the most valued guests, a matter amounting to a diplomatic exchange. And he noted that the esteem of the guest determined the status of the woman offered. Those persons held in low esteem might merit a maid or slave, women who may have been taken captive in a raid from another tribe.

The nature of this exchange requires more background. Among the Arikara, generosity was stressed at the expense of material wealth. A high ranking man was one who, above all else, was generous with his possessions and took care of the less fortunate. They could not conceive of it being otherwise. Recall that an Arikara told Tabeau (Abel 1939:135), a trader who was living with them at the time of the expedition's visit, that he was "wicked and foolish" because he did not give away his trade goods but "horded" them to be bartered for food and furs. Perhaps the Arikara regarded sex in a similar manner—something to be given away rather than to be withheld and hoarded. To do otherwise made the person both wicked and foolish. And for a host, the obligation to be generous might be particularly strong, including arranging opportunities for sexual relations.

Hospitality was but one of several for the reasons for sexual availability. There were others, including prostitution as well as establishing and maintaining trade relations.

Prostitution

Trudeau (in Smith 1936:567), who was quoted above, continued his thought, "and in consideration thereof [sexual favors] accept a few baubles or toys...This kind of commerce is carried on to a great length by our Canadian traders."

Prostitution, a form of trade, is said to be the earliest profession. If this statement is true, then the archaeological record might provide evidence for its existence, but prehistoric archaeology, at least, is frustratingly silent about this profession. The 19th century visitors of the Arikara, in contrast to prehistoric archaeologists, wrote much about the flesh trade and its details.

To flourish, prostitution requires four key elements. These elements include someone to negotiate the act ("pimps" or sex middle-men), women whose sexual services are available ("hookers" or prostitutes), materials exchanged for the sex (glass beads seemed to be the Arikara's favorite object of exchange), and men who are interested in these economic and sexual transactions ("johns" or clients). All four key elements are chronicled in the historic accounts.

The use of such terms as "pimp," "hooker," and "john" need to be examined in a spirit of useful and rational cultural relativism. Perhaps a parable best sets the stage. A possibly apocryphal Catholic missionary spent years among the Hopi, without making a single convert. As he departed, he asked one headman to explain the failure of the mission. "You scratch us where we do not itch." Reflect a moment on the current informal terms for members of the sex trade, and the moral freight usually carried by these words.

A pimp is considered a moral outcast, a man who lives as a parasite on the bodies and souls of abused women. He collects money, yet does no real work. The girls give him a Lincoln automobile; he gives them a black eye. A hooker is a woman beyond shame, who trades her most perfect gift – the secrets of her body, the privacy of her most private parts – for money to feed her pimp and her drug habit, both of which further degrade her. She is a fallen woman. No decent man would want her. A john is someone regarded with contempt by a hooker. She sees that he cannot, through his own charm or self-presentation, find a woman who will accommodate him willingly—and for free. She may be low on the social scale, but even she can look down on him. She can laugh with other hookers about the weaknesses and fetishes of her johns, of their strange thoughts and stranger desires, of their tiresome need to buy "admiration," of their wish to be told how virile and puissant they are.

Yet we may be blind to how much these pejorative thoughts and labels are creations of our Western European assumptions. We tend to think that cultures with gadgets have a monopoly on truth and correctness. We think of a fellow technocracy – Japan, for instance – and consider them to be "like us." Yet Japanese ideas on sex are wildly different from ours. Their sex shows, sex clubs, and sex comics are not only common-place, but are free of the shame and guilt that form a dark lining to our forays into the erotic. The meaning of a sex act has little connection to the stage of a culture's technical development.

The issue here is the *meaning* of Arikara sexual practices. Indeed, they might best be described in that cliché of gangster movies: "It's nothing personal; it's just business." The Arikara man who offers his most beautiful woman may have been potlatching. "Behold, I am a man of such substance that I am able to offer you this lovely woman. Not some worn-out captive, ruined by toil and suffering, but a plump, smiling woman, whose existence is a beneficence to us both." True hospitality. In the field of commerce, the Arikara had no gold or technical wonders to trade, but they could offer sex. An hour of sex for twenty strands of blue glass beads? If both parties are satisfied with the transaction, where is the harm? If the Plains Indians had

had Oprah or the Maury Povich show, would these women have sat sobbing, consumed in grief and shame? Not likely, unless they had been sold defective beads.

In brief, the Arikaras were traders. Sex for goods. Sex for status in their community. These transactions are ill defined by our standards and our moral judgments.

Sex Middlemen

Whatever the culture, arranging sex for hire often involves a male intermediary, one who arranges sexual liaisons with customers, ensures the prostitute's safety from clients and officials alike, and who profits from these and her labors. Although there is no indication of official obstacles to the 19th century sex trade, the Arikara middlemen mentioned in the historic accounts were the women's male relatives, most often their husband but not limited to him.

Trudeau (1914:461), the trader from St. Louis who lived with the Arikara during the summer of 1795, wrote "what is more, the fathers, brothers and even the husbands offer and take the youngest and most beautiful daughters, sisters and wives to the White Men for their diversion, in exchange for a few trifles which they receive." So, in addition to a woman's husband acting as the go-between, Trudeau noted that other male relatives, such as fathers or brothers for instance, might serve the same function.

Tabeau (Abel 1939:178), the caustic trader living with the Arikara when the Lewis and Clark Expedition visited in 1804, noted

> The most peculiar thing is that all goes on often in front of and even by order of a jealous husband.... [The husband] prostitutes her himself for a very small reward and it is seen that a wife has not yet been chastised for having failed in submission in like case.... This politeness is carried out every day among the Ricaras, and always the more readily in

the case of the whites; but infidelities, unavowed, are not always punished severely and the braves ordinarily content themselves with repudiating their wives. This is, often, only a momentary divorce. Besides, the intrigues are so common that they are generally made light of (Abel 1939:179-181).

The culturally modal behavior based on these historic accounts seems to be that male relatives arranged such liaisons, or at the least, they ignored the indiscretions. While cuckoldry is anathema to most Western men, the Arikara had a different perspective. Returning to Trudeau (1914:460), he observed that "The women never cause battles among them, for not having that kind of blind frenzy which we call love, they are not susceptible to jealousy, and do not know that passion. When a man dies, they say, he has not even his wives with him in the land of the dead, so that those who fight and kill each other for women are fools and mad men." So, according to the Arikara, not only can you not take your wealth with you, you can't take your wife—or wives—with you either.

The importance of husbands and other male relatives as middle men in the sex trade and their approval of such trade should be emphasized for the societal sanctions it implies. For an Arikara husband, arranging sexual liaisons was nothing to be ashamed of. Cuckoldry, on the other hand, might be a different matter. Where one condition blended into the other was a nebulous one, at least to the Western participants, and to them the situation was fickle.

Sometimes these interpretations and misunderstandings were caused by cultural differences. Other times, there were different causes. The best example of an apparent culturally-mediated sexual misunderstanding precipitating a catastrophic event was the situation leading to what has been called the "Arikara War."

Two decades after the Lewis and Clark visit, the Arikara villages were quickly becoming mere stop-overs for traders and trappers, not the terminal destination it had previously been for traders, such as Trudeau and Tabeau. St. Louis traders were pushing past the Arikara villages. Their goal was either to trade directly with tribes in the upper reaches of the Missouri River or do the trapping themselves. As a result, the Arikara's middleman position in the trade network, one established prehistorically and maintained into the early historic period, was eroding and unraveling. These developments and forces collided when William Henry Ashley and his men visited the Arikara villages in 1823. The following summary of this stop and events is based on Morgan's presentation (1953:59-77).

Ashley and his business partners organized the Rocky Mountain Fur Company to trap and trade on the Upper Missouri River. With a total force of approximately 90 men, his plan was to boat from St. Louis up the Missouri River to the Arikara villages. There he planned to split his force, part going overland to the Forks of the Missouri by riding horses purchased from the Arikara. The rest of the party was to continue their upriver journey to the trapping region by boat.

Ashley's party reached the Arikara villages in June 1823. Relations between the group and the Arikara were tumultuous—sometimes friendly, other times antagonistic. Following negotiations, an Arikara chief agreed to trade with Ashley's party. The party camped on a sandbar in front of the villages with boats anchored in the middle of the river, and goods ferried ashore as needed for trade.

Despite the shaky relations between the two groups, some of Ashley's men were fearless—or horny—enough to slip out of camp into the villages, presumably for some personal trading, most likely involving sex. Men, after all, have been known to take greater chances and to have done stupider things for sex.

One night a member of Ashley's party was killed while in the village and his body dismembered. We suspect that the murder was caused by a "trick" gone bad, our point being the tenuous nature of sexual relations as well as the shaky political and economic relations in which they were embedded during 1823.

The next morning there was an all-out attack on Ashley's sandbar camp. Despite onboard crew members' attempts to rescue on-shore party members, more than a dozen of Ashley's party were killed and others were wounded. The survivors floated down river, regrouping below. All because of a matter of sex?

What happened next was an early charade of American military might—but certainly not the last. Colonel Henry Leavenworth at Ft. Atkinson, now in eastern Nebraska, was notified of the slaughter. He organized his infantry and headed upriver, his command augmented along the way by Sioux and interested traders. The "Arikara War" was underway. The allied US phalanx arrived at the Arikara villages in mid-August 1823. Following an initial attack and engagement of the Arikara by the Sioux advance guard, the confrontation quickly devolved into a siege with artillery rounds lobbed into the Arikara villages with mixed results.

Negotiations between the military and the Arikara ensued. The Arikaras, claiming that an early artillery round had killed the primary troublemaker, were inclined to resolve the dispute with a truce. Col. Leavenworth, as part of the negotiations, demanded that the Arikara replace Ashley's lost goods, provide hostages as a sign of good faith, and in the future behave in a peaceful fashion. The Arikara equivocated, agreeing to some issues and contesting others.

As parleys continued from one day to the next, the Arikara, deciding that retreat was preferable to a negotiated peace, abandoned their villages one night, sneaking past Leavenworth's forces, escaping the surrounding US noose. The next morning, the villages were found vacant except an elderly woman who was too frail to travel, 50 dogs and one rooster. Col. Leavenworth claimed about 50 Arikara had been killed in the engagement. Thus, the Arikara War came to an inglorious end. The Arikara villages, the sites that now bear Col. Leavenworth's name, were vacated for approximately a year, while the Arikara wandered the Plains and visited other villagers, killing every white they could find. The Leavenworth villages were reoccupied the following year, and the Arikara continued residing there until 1832. Enough said about the Arikara War and the sexual relations that may have triggered it. Now we return to Arikara sex trade.

Other early 19th century chroniclers who indicated that some Arikara male relatives served as sex trade intermediaries reiterated Trudeau and Tabeau. Among those, Bradbury's account is notable.

Bradbury (1904:140), the botanist who visited the Arikara at the same time as Brackenridge, noted some details of the Arikara sex trade. "This evening [June 17, 1811] I judged that there were not fewer than eighty squaws, and I observed several instances wherein the squaw was consulted by her husband as to the *quantum sufficit* of the price; a mark of consideration which, from some knowledge of Indians, and the estimation in which their women are held, I had not expected." Bradbury indicated that male relatives—specifically husbands—were negotiating the deals, but, at least in some cases, husbands consulted their wives concerning acceptability of the negotiated price.

The political and economic power of Arikara women was often overlooked by less skilled white observers. Besides the relatively minor act of price setting, Arikara women were pivotal to Arikara culture—as women are in all cultures. They were the primary providers of family subsistence, being in charge of the entire horticultural process, from seed to bowl. It was their horticultural productivity that made intertribal and other outside trade possible; a reliable food surplus graciously provided by Arikara hosts was one of the things that drew visitors and kept them fed while trading. In addition, an older woman usually headed each earth lodge. It was her lodge that housed her extended family, including her daughters, sometimes even early into their marriages. Finally Arikara women conducted important ceremonies (Parks 2001:378). Not all travelers, however, were as observant as Bradbury.

Visiting the Arikara villages at the same time as Bradbury, barrister Brackenridge (1906:130) noted the same sex commerce, but with a different perspective. The "greater part of their females, during our stay, had become mere articles of traffic; after dusk, the plain behind our tents, was crowded with these wretches, and shocking to relate, fathers brought their daughters, husbands their wives, brothers their sisters, to be offered for sale at this market of indecency and shame...." Again, Brackenridge supports Trudeau and Bradbury's identification of pimps, but he differs in his assessment of the women's power and role in the transactions.

This gender- and Western-centrism extended well beyond the Lewis and Clark era. Only in the mid-20th century did women become involved in documenting women's perspectives and women's roles in Native Plains cultures. Until that time, few males provided reliable insights into female issues (cf. Weist 1980). So early 19th century accounts must be read with such limitations in mind.

With that caveat, finally there is an entry by Luttig, the clerk at Ft. Manuel Lisa in 1812-1813, which provides a glimpse of women's roles. He mentioned a husband offering his wife to the fort's occupants. In his entry for September 23, 1812, Luttig (1964: 81) noted "...another [Arikara] arrived to trade a horse and also his Wife, a handsome Squaw[.] he found trade for the horse but not for the Wife,..." As in all such cold, unsolicited sales transactions, one out of two ain't bad!

To summarize, the middlemen overseeing the Arikara sex trade were usually husbands, although other male relatives were mentioned in the historic accounts. They regulated and negotiated some portions of the sex trade. It is apparent that prostitution was socially condoned, even encouraged, at least by some male family members.

Prostitutes

Following months of plying the Missouri River, exposed to deprivations and tormented by mosquitoes, with little more than glimpses of women, the expedition's members rejoiced as they approached the Arikara villages. The Arikara were renowned as welcoming hosts—and there were always the Arikara women. The women's availability tempted members of the Lewis and Clark Expedition as they had other travelers for years and would for at least the next few decades. Sweetening the deal, some accounts claim that the Arikara women were particularly attractive. If this claim is indeed the case, it was not only their availability but their beauty that contributed to their popularity with white men.

For example, Sgt. Patrick Gass, a member of the Lewis and Clark Expedition, found the Arikara the most beautiful Indian women he had seen (in Lowry 2004:58). Perhaps as an understatement, Clark noted "Ricara women better looking than the Sioux" (in Lowry 2004: 58). And Ordway (1916:150) also noted the Arikara women's attractiveness in his entry for October 10, 1804: "Some of their women are verry handsome & clean &. C. &. C."

A few years after the Lewis and Clark Expedition, Brackenridge (1906:121) described the attractiveness of the women: "The women are much fairer than the men; some might be considered handsome any where;...." This assessment was the consensus in the early 19th century. And these conclusions were supported by portraits photographed 100 years later (Fig. 4).

There was a contrary perspective, however, one voiced by the acerbic resident trader who was living with the Arikara when the

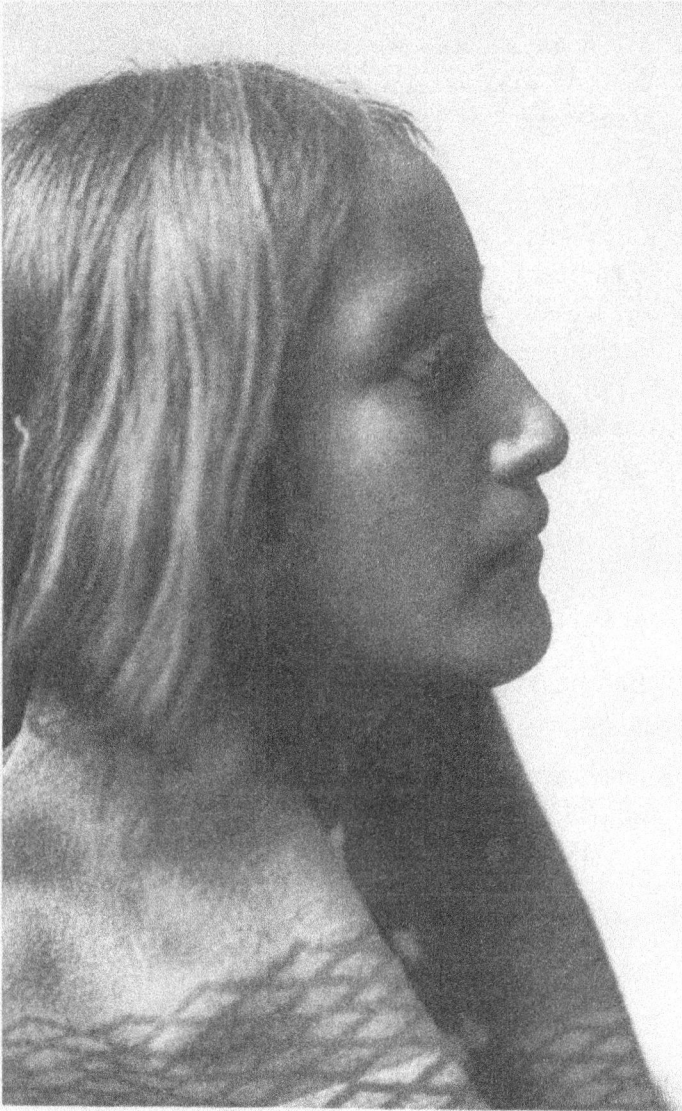

Figure 4. Edward Curtis's "Arikara Maiden" photographed in early 1900s showing beauty of Arikara women. (Used with permission of Northwestern University Library.)

expedition toiled up the Missouri River. Tabeau (Abel 1939:174) wrote

> As for the Ricara women, I have reason to believe that it is, in derision or in irony, that some travelers have called them the Circassians of the Missouri or else the present race has degenerated greatly. This is difficult to believe on seeing the old women. They are certainly the most ugly and have the advantage of surpassing all others in slovenliness. They generally have a color as of death, as far as one can judge through the layers of dirt, in which sweat or rain has traced lines. And I would not be accused of exaggeration here, if decency did not forbid detail, too repugnant. I shall only say that, after having eaten almost a year with the Ricaras, one ought not to be allowed to be fastidious or disgusted.

Never one to mince words, that Tabeau.

A comment on Tabeau's use of "Circassians" is worthwhile. Circassians were a people of the Caucasus Mountains in western Asia, whose women were claimed to be legendary beauties in the 18th and 19th centuries. So, comparing Arikara women with the Circassian women was high praise, whether it was intended directly or "in derision or in irony."

Were these polemic descriptions written about the same women? Perhaps they reflect the difference between short-time visitors and temporary residents. Perhaps they emphasize the differences between the visitors held in high esteem and travelers engaged in the sex trade on the one hand, and a trader of considerably lower status on the other. Perhaps Tabeau over-emphasized the older women, those who were probably not desirable in the sex trade as the younger ones. Perhaps other observers over-emphasized the younger more attractive women, ignoring the older less attractive ones.

Along these same lines, when one of the authors (PW) was working on the Crow Creek Indian Reservation, central South Dakota in 1978, a tribal member remarked to him about similar 20th century circumstances. White men, the tribal member complained, were much attracted to the tribe's youthful women, sometimes marrying and fathering children by them. But as the women aged and became less desirable, he continued, frequently the Indian women were divorced or abandoned. Then the women and their children often returned to the reservation, forced to rely on family and tribe for economic, emotional and social support. Youth and beauty, age and ugliness are arbitrary and culturally determined values that nevertheless have the impact of a 100-pound boulder.

Sailors have their mermaids—or manatees, depending on their state of mind. The thirsty have their mirage, consisting of sand and dust instead of water. Beauty is difficult to define and its perception varies with the circumstances. Some expedition members—sailors of the Missouri that they were—must have considered the Arikara women attractive, or at least attractive enough for their attentions and offered their meager belongings in exchange.

Beads

In addition to middlemen and prostitutes, for the sex industry to flourish there must also be a transfer of goods, the "trade" in sex trade. Although the expedition's accounts did not mention the items exchanged, other travelers did. What those accounts indicated was the most desirable objects were those exotic trifles the traders brought with them.

Trudeau (1914:460-461), the trader from St. Louis who lived with the Arikara during the summer of 1795, wrote "there is not one [Arikara woman] whose modesty is proof against a bit of vermillion or a few strands of blue glass beads;...." In another place Trudeau (Smith 1936:567) substitutes "blue ribbon" for the "blue beads" in

33

the previous quotation; we suspect the former is a typographical or translation error. Most likely both items were brought up the Missouri River or overland from Canada, and either would have been considered exotic and desirable goods, but beads were mentioned in other accounts and ribbon was not.

Bradbury (1904:140), the botanist who visited the Arikara villages in 1811, wrote " Mr. Hunt was kept in full employ during the evening in delivering out to them [the clients and prostitutes] blue glass beads and vermillion, the articles in use for this kind of traffic."

Barrister Brackenridge (1906:130), who visited the Arikara at the same time as botanist Bradbury, was more ambiguous about the items trafficked, although he noted the activity of the trade. He wrote "perhaps something may be attributed to the inordinate passion which had seized them [the Arikara] for our merchandise."

And seeming to confirm these assertions, Tabeau (Abel 1939: 178), a trader living with the Arikara when the Lewis and Clark Expedition visited in 1804, noted "It could be said that the latter [Arikara women] do justice to themselves and know the value of their favors, if their facility in granting them is any criterion. The most inflexible is not proof against a prize of vermillion and of twenty strands of beads. There are, nevertheless, a few prudes who greatly wish to pass for cautious ones; but surrender themselves, moreover, with discretion and secrecy...."

Although denigrating the Arikara women on the one hand, Tabeau was quick to note the value of the blue bead. Elsewhere, he (Abel 1939:176) described glass beads as being "as precious here as the porcelain among the natives of the Mississippi."

Incidentally, one of the authors (PW), while a Kansas University freshman, hand-counted the thousands of beads archaeologically recovered from the Leavenworth Site cemeteries by Bass. There were a total of 142,249 beads, the majority (131,972) being small blue "seed" beads (Bass et al. 1971:113-114, table 11). How many of these beads changed hands as part of sexual transactions and how many were passed in other transactions remains uncertain.

Blue beads and red pigment seemed to be the preferred items, but other goods were also involved, perhaps even blue ribbon and other cloth. Botanist Bradbury (1904:141) walked through an Arikara village accompanying Donald M'Kenzie, who was wearing a green surtout, a fashionable knee-length overcoat of the day. The coat attracted the attention the of Arikara women, apparently because its green cloth was a novelty to them. When the women offered him "favours" for small pieces of it, Bradbury joked that M'Kenzie's long knee-length coat might quickly become a spencer, a waistcoat, if the offers were accepted! Any of a variety of objects might be exchanged, it seems, but beads and vermillion were the most frequently mentioned in the accounts.

Based on these accounts, manufactured trade goods were employed in the sex trade, and some of the more unusual items may have been especially desirable. Whether the trade was as strings of beads (echoes of a New Orleans' Mardi Gras and cries of "show us yer mammaries!"), vermilion (perhaps anticipating the "painted ladies" of the more recent "Old" West) or cloth (more about that in a moment), the exchanges seemed to be frequent and socially sanctioned, sanctioned at least for the most part. Some of the Arikara visitors would give almost anything—and everything—for such favors. And some members of the expeditionary parties seemed more likely to be involved in the trade than others.

Clients

Laborers, boatman and French Canadians were especially enthusiastic customers of the trade. More exactly, they were the only customers, that is if the accounts by the well-to-do, literate chroniclers are to be believed.

Trudeau (1914:461), the trader from St. Louis who lived with the Arikara during the summer of 1795, wrote "Our young Canadians and Creoles who come here [Upper Missouri River] are seen everywhere running at full speed, like escaped horses, into Venus' country,...." What images—virile young men of ethnic extractions galloping through a sea of sex!

Much to the point, though not as colorful, botanist Bradbury (1904:140) wrote "The Canadians were very good customers...." This observation again implicates others and the underbelly members of the expeditions in the sex trade.

Barrister Brackenridge (1906:130) chimed in, supporting and elaborating Bradbury's account concerning the "Canadians." The boatmen of his party, Brackenridge claimed, were known for "their loose habits and ungovernable propensities" and were especially active in this trade. Brackenridge (1906:130) continued "The silly boatmen, in spite of the endeavors of the leaders of our parties, in a short time disposed of almost every article which they possessed, even their blankets, and shirts. One of them actually returned to camp, one morning entirely naked, having disposed of his last shirt—this might truly be called *la derniere chemissede l'amour*." Canadians, Creoles and boatmen (not mutually exclusive groups!) were those identified as the most frequent clients. In addition Brackenridge noted articles exchanged in the trade other than the usual beads and pigment; even clothing, blankets and nearly everything else was fair game.

The ardor of the Lewis and Clark Expedition's men must have been similar to that of Bradbury's Canadians and Brackenridge's boatmen a few years later, as well as Trudeau's Canadians and Creoles a few years before the expedition arrived. And the expedition's men had little contact with—even seen—few women since departing civilization months previously. There is no mention which of the expedition's men—or officers—may have engaged in sex, as might be expected of those whose pens told the stories.

There is a limitation to those accounts that identify the clients. The existing accounts were composed, for the most part, by elite members of the various expeditions, those who wrote and presented their observations. There are hints that a few chroniclers had sexual encounters. As an example, accounts indicate bedmates were offered to esteemed travelers, but none of the journalists indicated that they were involved, at least not in the "common" trade. On the other hand, none of the typical "johns," none of the Canadians or Creoles and few enlisted men, left written memoirs. If they had, they may have told a different story, one that implicated the elite members in sexual activities. The omission, if that is what it is, is unfortunate.

Not only is the dearth of "commoners'" perspectives on the sex trade unfortunate, there is yet another side to this story that is missing: the Arikara's perspectives. We are fortunate that one glimmer of the Arikara's perspectives survives, recorded by one of the travelers concerning his visit to the Arikara villages.

Barrister Brackenridge (1906:130) wrote "Seeing the chief one day in a thoughtful mood, I asked him what was the matter—'I was wondering,' he said, 'whether you white people have any women amongst you.' I assured him in the affirmative. 'Then,' said he, 'why is it that your people are so fond of our women, one might suppose that they had never seen any before.'"

This story is puzzling based on the other accounts indicating the willing Arikara participation in sexual activities. But the Arikara must have viewed the trade in much different contexts than the whites, the ones who wrote the documents.

The English- and French-speaking Euroamericans viewed the sex trade largely in an economic context. As the consummate traders, the Arikara knew how to sweeten the pot. Tit for tat, as it were. But the Arikara doubtlessly interpreted the trade in their cultural context, and as Brackenridge suggested, that included establishing and maintaining trade relationships. There were more ephemeral purposes, at least to our Western minds: transmitting spiritual power.

Transmit Spiritual Power

On a higher level, the Arikara, as some of the other Upper Missouri River Native Americans, believed that sexual intercourse transferred spiritual power between the participants and that transfer provided benefits to the individuals involved as well as their families, clans and communities.

In an earlier time, the Arikara held whites in high esteem, even to the point of veneration. This perspective, however, was quickly fading by the time of our early 19th century accounts. Trudeau (1914: 455), who lived with the Arikara during the summer of 1795, noted that the Arikara called EuroAmericans "White Men" or "Spirits." And these terms were not pejorative—at least not at that time. "It is said that formerly the Ricara nation held us in such veneration that they gave us a sort of worship, having certain festivals at which they offered us the choicest morsels, and even threw into the river robes, which had been dyed and dressed skins decorated with feathers, as a sacrifice to the white Man" (Fig. 5). These offerings and interpretations are similar to more recent Melanesian Cargo Cults, where Western manufactured goods were believed to be under magical control.

The classic cargo cults occurred when Melanesians were overawed by the material goods and wealth shipped by warring nations to that region during WW II. According to these native beliefs, their ancestors sent the war materiel, intended for them, their descendants,

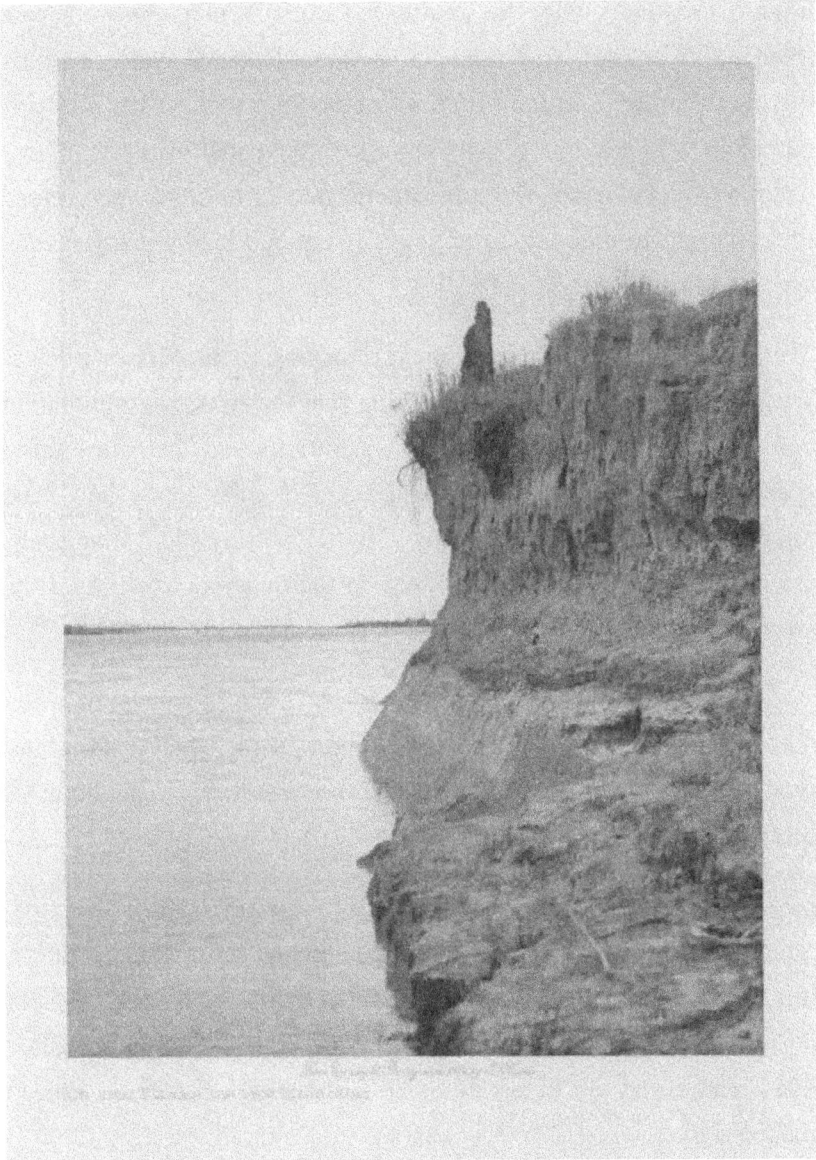

Figure 5. Edward Curtis's "On the Banks of the Missouri." The Missouri River was the lifeblood of the Arikara. (Used with permission of Northwestern University Library).

but it was intercepted by westerners and who used the goods for their own purposes. With the end of WW II and the cessation of hostilities among nations, troops vacated the South Pacific, leaving the Melanesians to wonder why the wealth was even further removed from them and their uses. To bring back the manufactured Western goods, the cargo culters cleared jungles to construct make-shift airstrips, complete with bamboo control towers and coconut headsets. These decoys were believed, via sympathetic magic, to ensure the return of their rightful manufactured goods (from Wikipedia, Cargo Cults, accessed December 20, 2006).

Leaving the Pacific Ocean and returning to the Missouri River, Trudeau continued his thought, noting that the Arikaras' veneration had turned to more pragmatic considerations and that the French-speakers, at least, were no longer revered. Familiarity had bred, among other things, contempt by 1795. Hopefully the Melanesians are no longer waiting for or relying on the material wealth that the strangers brought either.

Nevertheless, it was still early in the historic transition when members of the Lewis and Clark Expedition met the Arikara, and they may have profited from this veneration in the few years before it disappeared altogether.

These fantastic attributions of whites are not limited to sexual intercourse. Incredible stories abounded among the Arikara concerning the expedition. Tabeau (Abel 1939:200) noted that his Arikara host, "one of the most intelligent of the Ricaras," told him incredible tales concerning the Lewis and Clark Expedition's travails. Tabeau recorded two.

According to this Arikara chief, one of the expedition's obstacle's ascending the Missouri River, was a mouthless monster who acquired nutrients by inhaling meat smoke, primarily that of swans and vultures during the warm months. The monster's other bodily functions are not recorded, but they were doubtlessly remarkable as well.

The other obstacle the expedition was reputed to have overcome in its journey up the Missouri River was a tribe of Amazons (Abel 1939:200). In this tribe, boys were killed at birth, their genitals pulverized and the residue used to inseminate the Amazons, thus perpetuating the uni-sexed race. Girls had it better than boys, though not much better. The girls were placed in a cradle, hung in a tree, where they subsisted on the surrounding air. Once they had grown to an adequate size and acquired a level of maturity, the mothers returned to retrieve and enculturate their daughters in the Amazon ways.

These adventures echo those of Ulysses. No wonder expedition members were held in high esteem, even to the point of being "medicine." What woman—other than an Amazon, of course—could deny such men?

Of the expedition's men, York was considered the biggest "medicine" of all (Abel 1939:201). He was the first black person that the Arikara had seen, and York played to the amazed crowd, emphasizing his novelty. He claimed he was formerly a wild beast who consumed children until Clark had captured and tamed him. York's medicine was of such a magnitude that one Arikara husband arranged to have his qualities transmitted via sex to his wife in an earth lodge. While the act was being performed, the husband stood guard at the lodge's entrance to make sure that no one interrupted the transmission (Jackson 1978, 2:503).

Transmitting spiritual power through sex seems peculiar to many Westerners, but among humans sex rarely relates solely to its reproductive aspect. Among the myriad of non-reproductive reasons for sex, any excuse is probably as good as another. What is often odd—even perverted—to outsiders is the insiders' norm. With that situation in mind, what is known about Arikara-Arikara intramural sex?

Arikara Sex

Whatever the multiple and complex Arikara motivations for sexual relations with EuroAmericans may have been and whatever the proportion of Arikara involved, there appears to have been an active involvement of at least some Arikara women and some white men (as well as York) in sexual relations during the late 1700s and early 1800s. We suspect that similar activities occurred between the Arikara and members of other tribes, but those encounters are poorly documented. However there are a few accounts of Arikara-Arikara relations. Here we present topics related to Arikara sexual practices, including sex initiation of males, marriage patterns, extramarital affairs, sexual practices, and claims of incest.

Rather than the informal initiation to sexual relations that we experience in our culture ("catch as catch can," as it were), the Arikara had a more formal process, at least for males. First a little background is needed. Among an Arikara male's closest relatives were his brothers and maternal uncles. These male relatives were considered even closer than his own father, who came from a different kin group. As one indication of this close familial relationship among brothers and maternal uncles, an older brother's wife or a maternal uncle's wife typically initiated the younger brother or nephew in sex (Parks 2001: 378). All in the family, indeed! Sex education was one thing; however marriage was quite a different matter.

Trudeau (Smith 1936:566-568), the school master trader who lived with the Arikara in 1795, identified the preferred Arikara marriage pattern. According to him, a man had multiple wives, the wives being sisters—ideally at least. This form of marriage was so common among the Arikara that when a man married a family's oldest daughter, he often had the right to wed his wife's younger sisters as they came of age (Curtis 1909, 5:63). Termed "sororal polygyny," this marriage pattern has the advantages of sisters staying together in marriage and not being scattered from one hearth to others. These sisters knew one another their whole lives, and had similar economic dreams and social goals. Also recall that sisters shared half the same genes in common. Sisters took care of their sisters' children—as well as their own—and aided each other with onerous tasks. Brackenridge (1906:121) and Tabeau (Abel 1939:181-182) confirmed Trudeau's observations: polygyny was common. Arikara men sometimes had as many as four or five wives.

Such a marriage pattern works well if there is a "surplus" of females or a "deficit" of males, such as when male deaths exceed female deaths. That situation may have been the case. Brackenridge (1906:121) indicated that Arikara females exceeded Arikara males because warfare eliminated many males.

It is noteworthy that in many polygynous societies, only the wealthiest households are polygynous while the majority of relationships are one female-one male (monogamous) marriages. And in these societies, some males remain bachelors. It is unclear if such was the case among the Arikara. Perhaps Trudeau and Brackenridge noted polygyny among the prominent Arikara families while monogamy and bachelorhood were the rules among Arikara commoners. Monogamy, after all would have been the normal course of things from Trudeau's and Brackenridge's experience, and perhaps not as noteworthy as polygyny.

There were several other oddities that the chroniclers noted, oddities that from a cross-cultural perspective are actually not that unusual. If an Arikara husband should die, his brother became the new husband of the sister-based "harem." Again, this relationship emphasizes the closeness of brothers. This marriage pattern is a cross-culturally widespread practice known as the levirate. The levirate has the advantages of maintaining extended family relations following the husband's death. It ensures that wealth, offspring and kin are retained within the family and not diminished or debarred by out-marrying. Out-marrying would cause wealth and offspring to be distributed into a different family. Among the Arikara as many other traditional groups, family was first and foremost.

Trudeau (Smith 1936:566-568) noted that marriages—presumably both polygynous and monogamous marriages (although that was not stated explicitly)— were fragile, especially among young adults. There was much spouse changing until the age of 30 years. In middle age, marriages became more stable and tended to persist. Those trends were the ideal Arikara circumstances, at least as Trudeau saw them.

There were motivations for extramarital relations other than the youthful vigor chronicled in the historic accounts. Tabeau (Abel 1939:126-127) wrote that in July 1804 a Mandan-Arikara man "stole" a young Arikara woman fulminating "rival hordes" in the Arikara villages. The results were hardly inconsequential: two people were killed and others severely injured in the ensuing melee. Extramarital sexual relations were one thing, theft another.

The observer who wrote the most about these extramarital relations was Edwin Thompson Denig. Denig was born in Pennsylvania in 1812, became a fur trader, and was living on the Upper Missouri River by 1833, where he spent more than 20 years, most of that time at Fort Union. He died in Canada in 1858 (Ewers 1961:xiv-xxv), leaving a thick volume of writings describing the Upper Missouri River tribes.

Denig (1961:62) wrote

> Indians to be Indians must have war. Without it the young men have no occupation, no ambition, even if so disposed can do nothing to render their names and

characters conspicuous. He, be he ever so brave, is classed with the rest and seeks distinction in circumventing the young women. Instead of being a great warrior he desires to be known as a great rake, he has no other choice, and his time is devoted to this purpose. The same spirit is visible in the elderly men. Thrown upon their own resources, with much idle time, they seduce each other's wives. This being almost the only occupation of the males, their minds become so debased that in the end they make victims of their own blood relations. In conformity with the state of things the virtue of all their women is at the lowest ebb, and for sale to any person who is so unfortunate as to make application.

If Tabeau was acerbic, Denig was downright acidic.

Denig indicated that in the absence of war and given the impossibility of status acquisition through that traditional means, status, instead, could be achieved through sexual conquests. In addition to the obvious parallels of warfare accomplishments and sexual conquests, there is another sexual practice that is peculiarly unfamiliar to us and our Western ways of thinking. That notion is vulva capture.

Among some traditional Plains Indian tribes, female virginity included not only those women who had not had genital intercourse but extended to those women whose genitals had not been touched, fondled or violated by hand: vulva capture, it was called. There were exhaustive efforts on the part of some families to prevent vulva capture, even to the point of pinning young women's skirts to the earth or tying their legs together while they slept (Abel 1939:181). Although we Westerners might dismiss such fondling as comparatively innocent, Arikara women who experienced such sexual contact were no longer considered virgins. They had been violated. And males who achieved such "firsts" gained status in a manner comparable to counting coups (Mickelson 1932; Powers 1986).

Back to Denig, he implied that at least some Arikara sexual license was a recent phenomenon, following the mid-19th century reduction in warfare. Sex was substituted, he claimed, when other, more traditional means of male social climbing were no longer available. Unfortunately for 21st century scholars, Denig had little first-hand knowledge of the Arikara (Ewers 1961:xxxiii) and his tenure in the region began after the Arikara abandoned the Leavenworth Site. There are some indications that Denig may have presented a distorted view of the Arikara.

Concerning incest, Denig (1961:53) wrote "Many of the Arikara families sleep indiscriminately together, the father beside the daughter, the brother with the sister, and this is the only nation among whom incest is not regarded as either disgraceful or criminal." Denig was not alone. Tabeau noted intrafamily sexual relations. He claimed to have observed brother-sister sexual relations (Abel 1939:181).

Across all cultures, the most eschewed sexual relationships are those involving close relatives. Incest taboos are known in all cultures and there are few—if any—groups that violate them. No known culture, after all, is completely promiscuous. All societies have rules and expectations concerning sexual behavior.

This statement impugns Denig's credibility, as well as Tabeau's. Why would Denig have made such denigrating remarks? Was it a lack of familiarity with the Arikara? Or was it his Assiniboin wives, hailing from a tribe who were long-term enemies with the Arikara? We suspect that it may have been a combination of the two.

So, among the 19th century Arikara, as all peoples, sexual relations had meanings beyond the biological, mundane and tangible—ramifications that few early travelers understood. Whites interpreted sexual relations in a variety of ways, but typically within the context of their own culture's perceptions and mores.

Summary

In this chapter we considered the reasons for the sexual license that many of the historic accounts noted. The first reason was hospitality by a group well-versed in the nuances of trade. One aspect of that trade was institutionalized prostitution. Components of the Arikara sex trade included male relatives acting as intermediaries in the transactions, trade goods (including glass beads and red pigment) often being bartered, attractive young women in the offing, and willing clients among the trappers, traders and travelers.

On the Arikara's part, there were a number of concepts and behaviors that seemed particularly odd to the Western observers. Arikara believed that powers could be transmitted through the sexual act from one participant to another, and from one of those participants to yet a third party. Also the Arikara had formalized sex education more than a century and a half before US public schools accepted the challenge. This hands-on training involved the male adolescent initiate's brother's wife or maternal uncle's wife. In addition, the Arikara practiced sororal polygyny and the levirate, customs that must have perplexed the early 19th century observers. The possibility of Arikara incest has been considered.

Whatever meaning comes from sexual activity, regardless of the cultural lens it is viewed through, there are always fundamental facts of biology: sexual activity may lead to conception as well as transmission of disease. These are the issues considered in the next chapter.

4. The Wages of Licentious Sex

The sexual contact and frequency claimed for the Arikara has predictable outcomes, including extramarital pregnancies and venereal diseases.

Concerning the first of the two outcomes, fecundity of the Lewis and Clark Expedition members is rumored, particularly by York among the Mandan. There are also rumors of offspring fathered by other expedition members. There was a Nez Perce man, for instance, named Daytime Smoker who claimed to be the son of Capt. William Clark, fathered by him during the expedition's sojourn. Daytime Smoker was photographed in 1867 and that image is on file at the Wisconsin Historical Society (Figure 6).

Other than offspring, another outcome of such sexual contacts was infectious diseases. Their effects were noted in some of the historic accounts, including that by Clark. The month after their visit with the Arikara, when they were beginning winter near the Mandan, Clark's journal entry for November 12, 1804, indicated "3 men Sick with the [blank]." The blank resulted from a crossed-out word, apparently marked through by Biddle (Moulton 2002, 2:233), an early

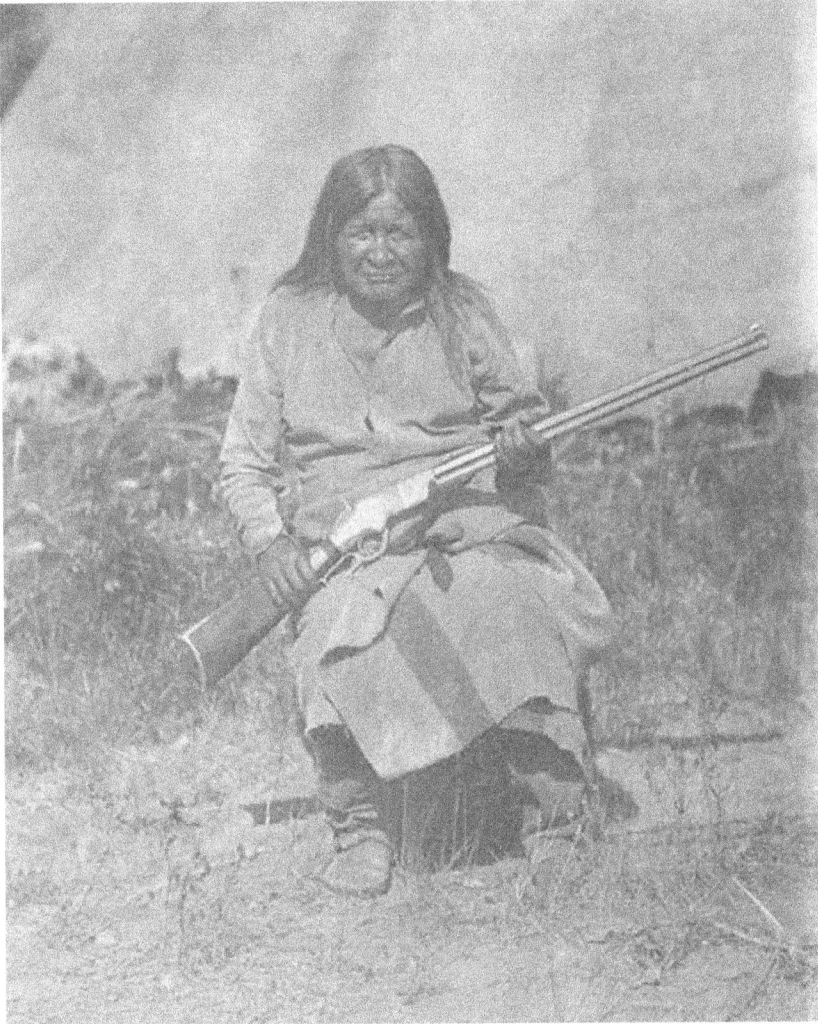

Figure 6. Daytime Smoker, a Nez Perce who claimed to be the son of William Clark, fathered during the time the expedition spent with that tribe. (From Wisconsin Historical Society, image WHi-6541; used with permission).

editor of the Lewis and Clark journals. This entry indicated that venereal disease symptoms were occurring among the expedition's men and it is likely that the disease was acquired from the Arikara.

Our argument for expedition members contracting venereal disease from the Arikara is shown as a timeline (Fig. 7). But first we present the facts, then the interpretations.

MONTH		JOURNAL ENTRIES	EXPECTED SEQUENCE
1804	OCTOBER	2nd - Arrive Arikara 4th - Depart Arikara	Assumed infection
	NOVEMBER	12th - Journal notes VD	Expected date of chancre
	DECEMBER		Chancre persists
1805	JANUARY		
		14th - Journal notes VD	Expected onset of secondary
		21st - Journal notes VD	syphilis signs and symptoms

Figure 7. Timeline relating Lewis and Clark Expedition's Arikara visit and appearance of venereal disease symptoms among expedition members.

The facts include dates and notations. The expedition arrived at the Arikara villages on October 2, 1804 and departed October 4, possibly accompanied or joined by two young Arikara women. On November 12, five weeks after departing the Arikara, Clark wrote that three men were ill and additional venereal disease symptoms were recorded eight weeks later, on January 14, 1805 as well as the following week (see Lowry and Willey 2007 for references). This chronology coincides with the expected time of onset and reoccurrence of syphilis symptoms.

The interpretation of syphilis employs the accounts just presented and the expected sequence of syphilitic sequelae. Following initial exposure, 3 weeks is the modal incubation period for the primary symptoms of syphilis (chancres), although the time of onset is variable, ranging from 2 to 10 weeks. Chancres, once they appear, typically persist for 3 to 6 weeks. Following the chancre, there is a period of quiescence, lasting for 6 to 8 weeks. Then the secondary symptoms—skin and membrane rashes—appear, these lasting 2 to 4 more weeks. Note that the sequence and timing of the expedition's men's ailments coincide with those expected of syphilis (Fig. 7).

In this chapter, we provide historic accounts of venereal disease among the Arikara, including those of the expedition members as well as others' observations. In a subsequent section of this chapter, we present what was known about disease, in particular venereal disease, in Lewis and Clark's time. Then we consider the clinical courses of syphilis and other venereal diseases based on our modern understanding.

Accounts of Venereal Disease from the Lewis and Clark Expedition

What was known of disease in 1800? While the sciences of anatomy and surgery had made considerable progress over the centuries, the theories of communicable diseases wallowed in a miasma of medieval beliefs, interwoven with astrology. Today, we have several useful theories: tissues are divided into individual cells; disease is caused by bacteria, viruses, and tiny parasites; the hormone-secreting glands control many bodily functions.

In Lewis and Clark's time, however, the four humors governed medical thought. The humors were blood, phlegm, yellow bile, and black bile, each having a different effect on the person. A dominance of blood yielded a sanguine personality; excess blood caused a plethora that required bleeding by the doctor. Excess phlegm yielded the indolence of the phlegmatic personality. Under the sway of yellow bile, a choleric man was quick to anger; a surfeit of black bile caused depression. (Melancholy = melan [black] + chol [bile]). In a complex series of concepts, the four humors were related to the four elements (fire, air, earth, and water) and to the conjunctions of the dominant planets.

How were these theories useful to Lewis and Clark, treating sick men 2,000 miles from the nearest physician? The answer is: they were not. There were, however, some concepts that were useful to them.

When the expedition visited the Arikara villages, some aspects of venereal diseases were well known by Western medicine. Two venereal diseases were widely recognized by the early 1800s: syphilis and gonorrhea. Benjamin Bell distinguished the two diseases in 1793, the decade before the expedition's journey. Despite this distinction, the diseases were often considered merely two different manifestations of the same illness.

Although Clark's entry concerning venereal disease does not specify which disease the men contracted, Lewis and Clark were aware of the two diseases' distinctions. Lewis, for instance, while among the Shoshones distinguished between "ganaraehah" and "Louis Venerae" (Chuinard 1979:312).

A few comments on spelling are in order. Comparable to other entries in these explorers' journals, spelling of the venereal diseases—when identified at all—was arbitrary and whimsical. Standardized US spelling was in its infancy during the early 19th century—literally while the expedition was underway. Noah Webster's first dictionary, *A Compendious Dictionary of the English Language*, was published in 1806, followed by *An American Dictionary of the*

English Language published in 1828. Standardized spelling would have to wait until the expedition returned. Lewis and Clark, after all, had a continent to explore. They also had diseases to describe and treat, whatever their standardized spelling might be.

Correct spelling or not, Lewis made a similar distinction between syphilis and gonorrhea among the Chinooks (Biddle cited in Chuinard 1979:342) and possibly also among the Mandans, where he noted "both sorts of vl [sic.]" (Biddle in Chuinard 1979:263). Differentiation between the two diseases was significant and more than an academic exercise. The afflicted required different medical treatments depending on the disease they had.

The standard, mainstream treatment of syphilis in the 19th century was gum of guaiacum (a genus of New World woody plant) and low doses of mercury over long periods. The usual mercury treatment involved oral administration as well as salves placed on the primary lesion. Some physicians recommended bleeding before mercury treatments, but it is unclear if the captains followed this procedure. Mercury treatments continued until the patient's gums became sore and inflamed, and the mouth watered excessively. Treatment was discontinued until the resulting gingivitis diminished. Then treatment recommenced and continued until the disease was cured, or at least the symptoms disappeared (Chuinard 1979:134). Treatment with mercury was probably ineffective for the unfortunate syphilis victim. The ineffectiveness of the treatment led to the adage, "A night with Venus, a lifetime with mercury."

Lewis and Clark must have been familiar with syphilis and its treatment. Both captains had previous military experience and association with young men. In addition, Lewis had medical instruction from Benjamin Rush, a leading physician of the day, in Philadelphia. And both captains had the availability of physician Antoine Francois Saugrain in St. Louis the winter before they began their journey.

Did the captains anticipate venereal disease during the expedition? Definitely. Lewis's famous Philadelphia shopping list included five medications for venereal disease: sugar of lead, calomel, copaiba, and mercury ointment, as well as Dr. Rush's pills, which contained mercury. Lewis also purchased four pewter penis syringes intended for treating gonorrhea (Lowry 2004:35-45).

Not until the early 1900s was a more reliable treatment for syphilis developed than the mercury-based one. It was salvarsan, an arsenic compound. This treatment emerged about the same time that the causative agent of syphilis was identified (the bacterium *Treponema pallidum*) and the definitive Wasserman blood test was developed to identify the presence of *T. pallidum*. Penicillin, the first truly effective medical course, became available only in the 1940s. (Ortner 2003:278-297; Aufderheide and Rodriguez-Martin 1998:157-164; Powell and Cook 2005:20-24).

Gonorrhea was treated differently than syphilis. To treat the common symptoms of gonorrhea— burning and difficulty while urinating, or a urethral discharge—the urethra was irrigated with solutions. As mentioned above, such eventualities were anticipated for the journey as indicated by the expedition's medical shopping list: four penis syringes and medicines purchased in Philadelphia. Syringes were used to flood the urethra with medicines. Such medicines included Saccharum saturni (sugar of lead, lead acetate) and balsam of copaiba, which were listed on the expedition's medical inventory (Chuniard 1979:159), as well as saltpeter (Chuinard 1979: 156). Saltpeter, if its reputation is to be believed and it was used early enough, may have nullified the necessity of venereal disease medicines altogether!

Other Accounts of Venereal Disease among Arikara

The Lewis and Clark expeditionary force had company in contracting and noting venereal illnesses among the Arikara. There were four contemporary accounts describing venereal diseases among early 19th century Arikara.

Trudeau (1914:460-461), the school teacher-trader from St. Louis who lived with the Arikara during the summer of 1795, wrote "Our young Canadians and Creoles who come here...rarely emerge without being afflicted with the ills which are almost inseparably connected with it, for the *foul distemper* [emphasis added here] is more common here than the small pox is in the northern countries of Canada." In another account (Smith 1936:567), Trudeau speaks more directly of the illness: "The consequence of these libertine manners is the venereal disease." He identified in the second quotation what he called the "foul distemper" in the first quotation more exactly as venereal disease. In both sources, note that Trudeau identified the illness in the singular, not plural, a point discussed in a moment.

In his section titled "The Ricaras," Tabeau (Abel 1939:151), the acerbic trader living with the Arikara when the Lewis and Clark Expedition toiled up the Missouri River in 1804, wrote "Strangers, like the natives of the region, enjoy perfect health and I believe that, were it not for accidental illnesses and especially the venereal diseases, one would be ill only to die." By "accidental illnesses" we believe that he was probably referring to the injuries and trauma often associated with warfare and day-to-day life in a violent region. In addition, he observed that venereal diseases were marked and frequent contrasted with other illnesses, which, with the exception of the previously mentioned accidental ones, he wrote were infrequent.

Note that Tabeau, contrasted with the previous quotation from Trudeau, used the plural noun, suggesting that there was one venereal disease present. He was inconsistent on this matter. When Tabeau continued discussing venereal disease several chapters later, he used the singular noun (Abel 1939:183): "The venereal disease makes terrible ravages here and, from the moment it attacks a man, it makes more progress in eight days than elsewhere in five or six weeks." So, in this quotation, Tabeau claimed that there was but one disease and it was a pernicious one.

Botanist Bradbury (1904:180), in an entry made in July 1811, three or four weeks after visiting the Arikara, noted that "at least two-thirds of our Canadians" contracted venereal disease, which Bradbury referred to as the "unpleasant consequence" of sexual relations in one place and "this evil" in another without more exact details concerning the disease or diseases involved.

The disease or diseases present among the Arikara in the early 19th century are difficult to identify from the historic records alone. Although most documents remain ambiguous on the point, there are a couple of accounts that are more explicit.

David Thompson was a late 18th century and early 19th century Canadian trader. While visiting the nearby Mandan (Fig. 1) in 1797-1798, he noted that the men who had traveled with him from Canada had contracted "siphylis" (Thompson 1916:234). This identification, however, was made before the distinction between gonorrhea and syphilis was well established and must be considered suspect. The disease could have been gonorrhea. Thompson was almost certainly unaware of the difference, despite the cutting-edge distinctions between the diseases having just been established.

F.V. Hayden (Fig. 8) wrote the 19th century account that most definitively identified the Arikara venereal disease. He was a trained physician, having graduated from the Albany Medical College in 1853 and served as a surgeon during the Civil War (http://en.wikipedia.org/wiki/F.V._Hayden; accessed June 29, 2006). He wrote (Hayden 1862:355) "both young and old are often more or less tainted with syphilitic diseases." Note that he specifically refers to syphilis by name, but then complicates the diagnosis

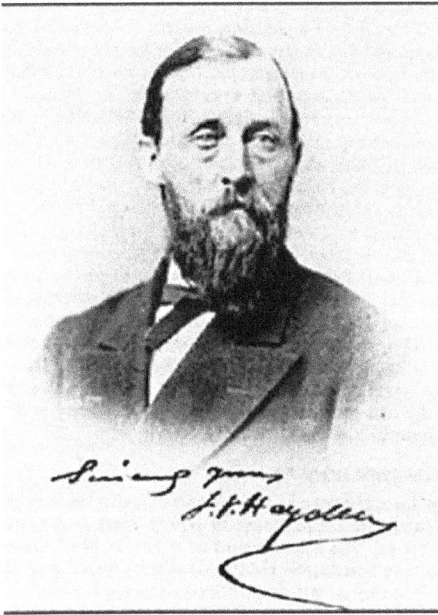

Figure 8. F.V. Hayden, physician, who visited the Upper Missouri River Region in the mid-1800s and identified "syphilitic diseases" among the Arikara. (From Wikipedia, accessed January 2, 2007).

using the plural noun, "diseases." The protean manifestations of syphilis may be the basis for his use of this plural noun.

Early physicians noticed that any part of the body could be ravaged by syphilis, so it appeared as a cluster of myriad symptoms. The victim could manifest tetters or morphia or rupia or insanity or tinnitus or transient blindness or running sores. But whatever its expression, you still had syphilis—the "syphilitic diseases."

Hayden also used "tainted" to describe the spread of the disease among the Arikara. We believe he meant that victims showed the depredations of disease, perhaps manifesting rot or corruption. It must be noted, however, that Hayden saw the Arikara decades after the Lewis and Clark Expedition and long after the Arikara abandoned the Leavenworth villages, so the applicability of his disease identification to the earlier Arikara is questionable.

It is noteworthy that Hayden's quotation is virtually identical to that attributed to Edwin Thompson Denig, the long-term Upper Missouri River trader mentioned in the previous chapter. Concerning the Arikara, Denig (1961:54) wrote "Both young and old of either sex are more or less tainted with the venereal disease." Note the similarities between this quotation and Hayden's. The few differences between Hayden and Denig's accounts were that Denig's version implicated both sexes, and Hayden's account indicated the specific venereal "diseases" (syphilis) present. Most likely Hayden plagiarized Denig's writing, providing a more exact identification of the disease in his slightly modified version.

Denig's (1961:54) account continued "This [venereal disease] also makes its appearance in their children in the form of scrofula and other cutaneous eruptions, and these know no end. The iniquities of the parents are literally visited upon their children even to the third and fourth generations." Denig seemed to be indicating the presence of congenital syphilis, although "scrofula" usually indicated tuber- culosis of the neck's lymph glands, which venereal diseases rarely cause.

When the early travelers described venereal diseases, did they mean syphilis or gonorrhea? The question was close to meaningless to them, because most of them were unclear as to the differences, and many medical authorities were equally confused, believing the diseases were different manifestations of the same illness. This con- fusion persisted until the late 19th century. By extrapolation, however, we can make a retrospective identification.

Gonorrhea in males is manifested frequently by a urethral dis- charge, often associated with painful urination. Without a careful examination of the affected parts, an examiner would see no visible disease. In females, the infection is even less manifest, usually being confined to the cervix and Fallopian tubes.

In contrast with gonorrhea, syphilis has visible surface lesions. There are the penile and vulva chancres during the primary stage, the measles-like rash of the secondary stage, and, in the late stage, the multitude of lumps, bumps, sores, excrescences, scabs, tetters, morphia, rupias, and oozing skin ulcers, not to mention collapsed nasal cartilages, erosions of the skull, and inflammations of the shins. In brief, syphilis is visual, while gonorrhea is more tactile. When a 19th century observer *saw* venereal disease, it was almost certainly syphilis, not gonorrhea.

In conclusion, there was venereal disease—or perhaps venereal diseases—present among the Arikara by the late 1700s and early 1800s. In addition to Lewis and Clark, there were four other relatively independent accounts of venereal disease among the Arikaras. The specific disease or diseases the Arikara carried, however, were not identified in the accounts from the early 1800s, although decades later, a formally trained physician (Hayden) identified their ailment as the "syphilitic diseases."

Today's understanding and treatment of diseases are very different than they were 200 years ago. Before looking at the 19th century Arikara skeletons and our 21st century interpretations of them, we need to delve into modern perspectives of the venereal diseases.

Clinical Expression of Venereal Diseases

There are many sexually transmitted diseases that may have affected the 19th century Arikara and their consorts. The best known and most debilitating venereal diseases recognized now are chlamydia, herpes, HIV/AIDS, gonorrhea, and syphilis. Today those diseases are distinguished based on the germ theory, which claims that infections are caused by distinct and different microorganisms, even if the symptoms of the diseases are similar. In this section, the major venereal diseases that affect the skeleton are described, including the causative organism, initial symptoms, and in the subsequent section, we consider the long-term effects of two venereal diseases on bones.

Infection with the organism *Chlamydia trachomatis* results in chlamydia. The first symptoms, which usually occur 1 to 3 weeks after initial infection, are often mild. Females may experience an abnormal vaginal discharge or burning sensation while urinating. Males, in turn, may experience a urethral discharge or a burning sensation while urinating. Untreated, long-term chlamydia may result in Reiter's Syndrome, which may cause arthritis in some individuals. The joints most frequently involved in Reiter's Syndrome are the knee, ankle and foot, although joints of the hands and spine may also be affected. Such arthritic changes are often non-diagnostic, ambiguous, and Reiter's Syndrome is likely to be confused with other forms of arthritis (Aufderheide and Rodriguez-Martin 1998: 104-105).

The most frequently identified venereal diseases in the 19th century were syphilis and gonorrhea. Chlamydia and the other venereal diseases were not identified until years later.

Gonorrhea is caused by the bacterium *Neisseria gonorrhoeae*. The earliest symptoms of gonorrhea usually occur 2 to 5 days after infection and initially involve soft tissue of the urethra. Females may experience a burning sensation while urinating or an unusual vaginal discharge. Males may experience a burning sensation while urinating or a urethral discharge. Many infected people, however, are asymptomatic and do not realize they have contracted the disease. Untreated, gonorrhea may spread to the prostate, cervix, and continue up the reproductive tract to other organs. In addition to reproductive structure involvement, gonorrhea tends to cause symptoms similar to synovitis, causing inflammation along the tendon sheaths.

The best-known sexually transmitted disease during the 19th and early 20th centuries was venereal syphilis. Venereal syphilis, caused by *Treponema pallidum*, comes in two forms. Acquired venereal syphilis (also known as lues) is transmitted by sexual contact.

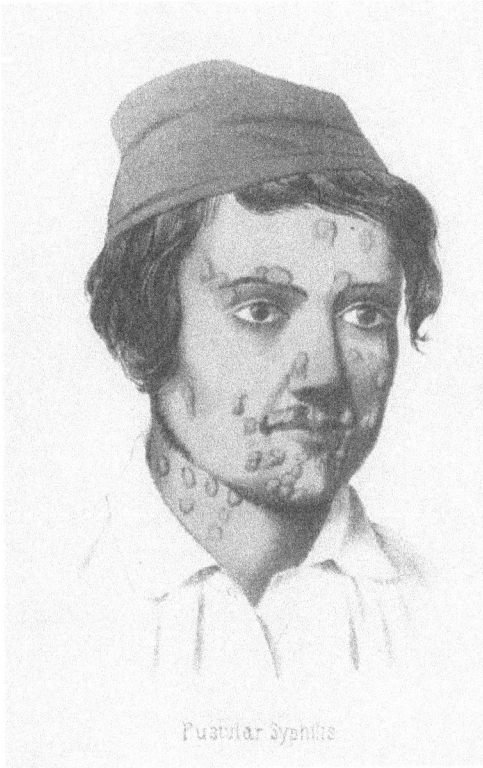

Figure 9. Mid-19th century lithograph of syphilitic male victim showing secondary stages of disease. (From Durkee 1866 *A Treatise on Gonorrhea and Syphilis*).

Following an incubation period, averaging 3 weeks but varying from 10 days to 10 weeks, a painless chancre erupts, usually on the genitals, indicating the site of inoculation and the first stage of the disease. Following the chancres' healing after 3 to 6 weeks and migration of the spirochetes to the lymph glands, there is a period of quiessence while the microbes spread through much of the body. Acquired venereal syphilis' second phase is a skin rash and inflammation of mucus membrane, usually 6 to 8 weeks after appearance of the chancre (Fig. 9). Secondary phase acquired syphilis usually lasts 2 to 6 weeks, followed by another period of quiesence. Among the untreated, the tertiary phase is marked by the invasion of any of a variety of organs, including those of the skeletal, cardio-vascular and nervous systems, usually 1 to 10 years after initial infection. The indications of acquired venereal syphilis, however, are highly variable,

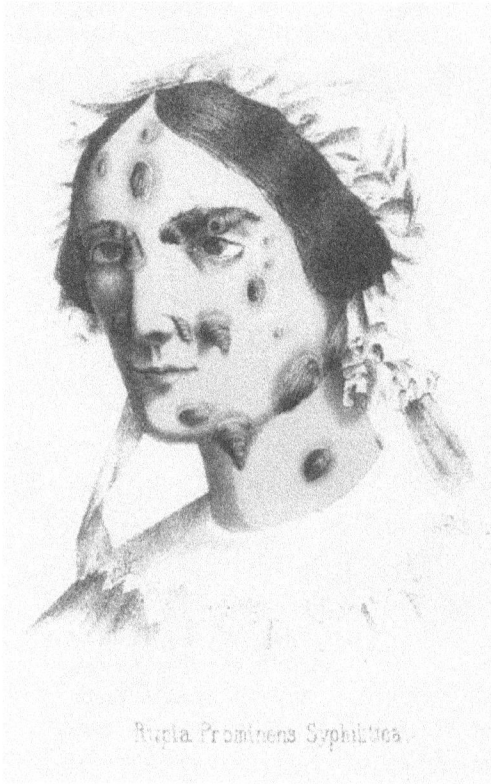

Ruia Prominens Syphilites.

Figure 10. Mid-19th century lithograph of syphilitic female victim showing idiosyncratic disease manifestations. (From Durkee 1866 *A Treatise on Gonorrhea and Syphilis*).

leading earlier clinicians to call it the "great imitator" because of the disease's ability to mimic the symptoms of many other diseases (Fig. 10). To make matters worse, there are also infected persons who do not display symptoms.

In addition to the clinical expression of acquired venereal syphilis, it is important to understand acquired venereal syphilis' epidemiology, that is, the distribution of the disease in a population. The peak of initial acquired venereal syphilis infection is in early adulthood. That age is when people are sexually most active, usually from 15 to 30 years, the disease peaking between 20 to 25 years. The rate of acquired syphilis infection in pre-antibiotic days was estimated to be between 5 to 10% in urban areas (Ortner 2003:278-297; Aufderheide and Rodriguez-Martin 1998:157-164; Powell and Cook 2005:20-24), although the frequency of some special groups had much higher frequencies. California Civil War troops, for instance, had rates as high as 50% (Murphy 1985).

The other form of the disease is congenital venereal syphilis. It is transmitted from the infected mother through the placenta to the fetus, most frequently occurring when the mother is in the early, proliferating phase of acquired venereal syphilis infection. The fetus is most vulnerable to infection during the second and third trimesters, resulting in 50% fetal mortality.

A fetus that survives syphilitic infection may express one of two kinds of congenital syphilis: early or late manifestations. The early form of congenital syphilis occurs between birth and 2 to 5 years. It involves rarefaction of the proximal tibia metaphysis, although osteochrondritis may occur there or at other anatomical locations. In addition to osteochondritis, osteomyelitis or periostitis may occur.

The late form of congenital venereal syphilis occurs after 2 to 5 years of age and has some characteristics similar to the skeletal lesions of acquired venereal syphilis. It includes soft, spongy localized defects (gummatous lesions) and saber shins (lower legs that bow forward). In addition to these familiar lesions, the late form of congenital syphilis may cause facial growth alterations resulting in a "saddle-shaped" nose and facial area, as well as Hutchinson's incisors and mulberry molars in 30-50% cases (Aufderheide and Rodriguez-Martin 1998:164-168; Powell and Cook 2005: 24-31)

Skeletal Expressions of Venereal Syphilis and Gonorrhea

The previous clinical information on venereal diseases provides a context, sequence and soft tissue perspective on skeletal involvement of the diseases. This foundation is now applied to the skeletal system in this chapter and then extended to the 19th century Arikara skeletons in the next chapter.

Some venereal diseases, as many chronic diseases, leave skeletal alterations, but these skeletal lesions are often ambiguous, diagnostic of many different diseases, and so cannot be used to identify a specific disease. The best osteologist, for instance, might not be able to differentiate the skeletal manifestations of AIDS from that of osteoporosis. Syphilis is an important exception to the ambiguous expressions of diseases on the skeletons. It is an infection capable of leaving diagnostic marks on the skeleton. Gonorrheal skeletal involvement is more ambiguous, however.

Gonorrhea may cause skeletal lesions. Ortner and Putschar (1985:399) note one skeletal alteration associated with gonorrhea: septic arthritis. Septic arthritis, however, is also associated with organisms other than gonococci. Gonococcal arthritis is distinguished from the other septic arthritises by usually being present at more than a single joint. Skeletal involvement, when it does happen, usually effects knees and ankles, and less frequently the sternoclavicular, intervertebral, temporo-maxillary, and sacro-iliac joints. These changes are more frequent in males than females.

Contrasted with other venereal ailments as well as many other nonvenereal diseases, the skeletal indicators of venereal syphilis are relatively distinctive. With venereal syphilis, skeletal lesions may be from either the acquired or congenital forms of the disease.

Skeletal manifestations of long-term acquired venereal syphilis occur in 10 to 20 percent of those in the tertiary phase of the disease (Steinbock 1976:109). The spirochete prefers cooler locations of the body, thus the coolest parts are typically where it is manifested. The spirochete targets and alters the skull vault, face and some portions of the skeleton below the skull. The most distinctive skeletal lesions associated with tertiary acquired syphilis are dramatic bone lumps and bumps on the skull vault (caries sicca). They occur most frequently on the forehead, top and sides of the cranial vault (Fig. 11).

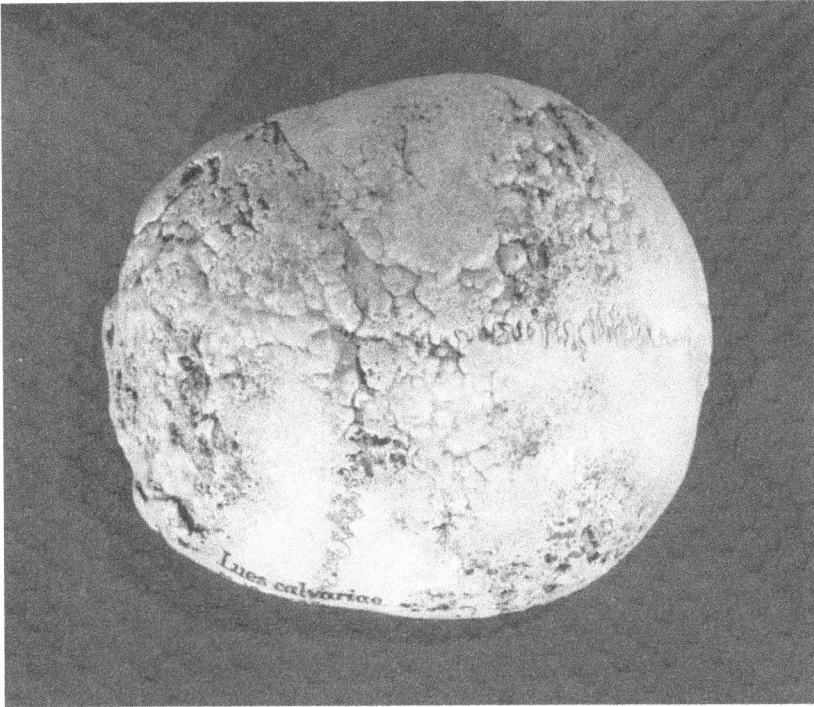

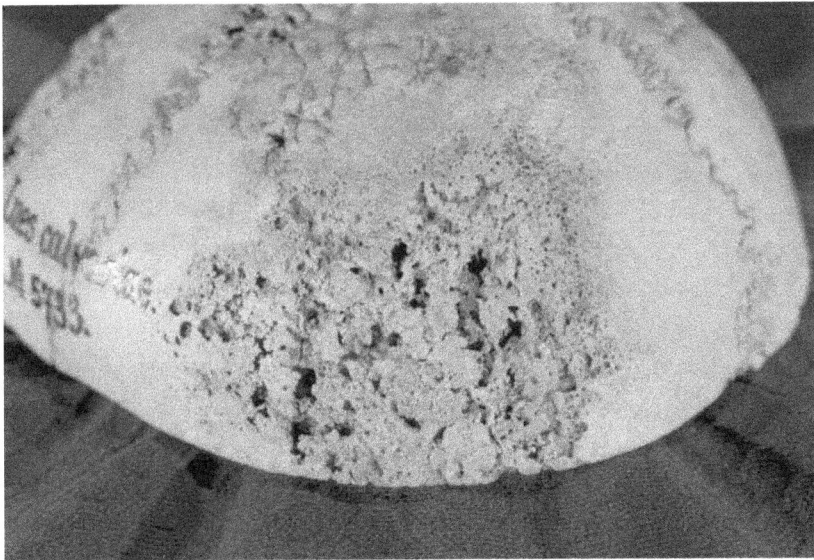

Figure 11. Skull vault showing caries sicca caused by tertiary syphilis. (From Donald J. Ortner, images 002-369 and 002-371; used with his permission).

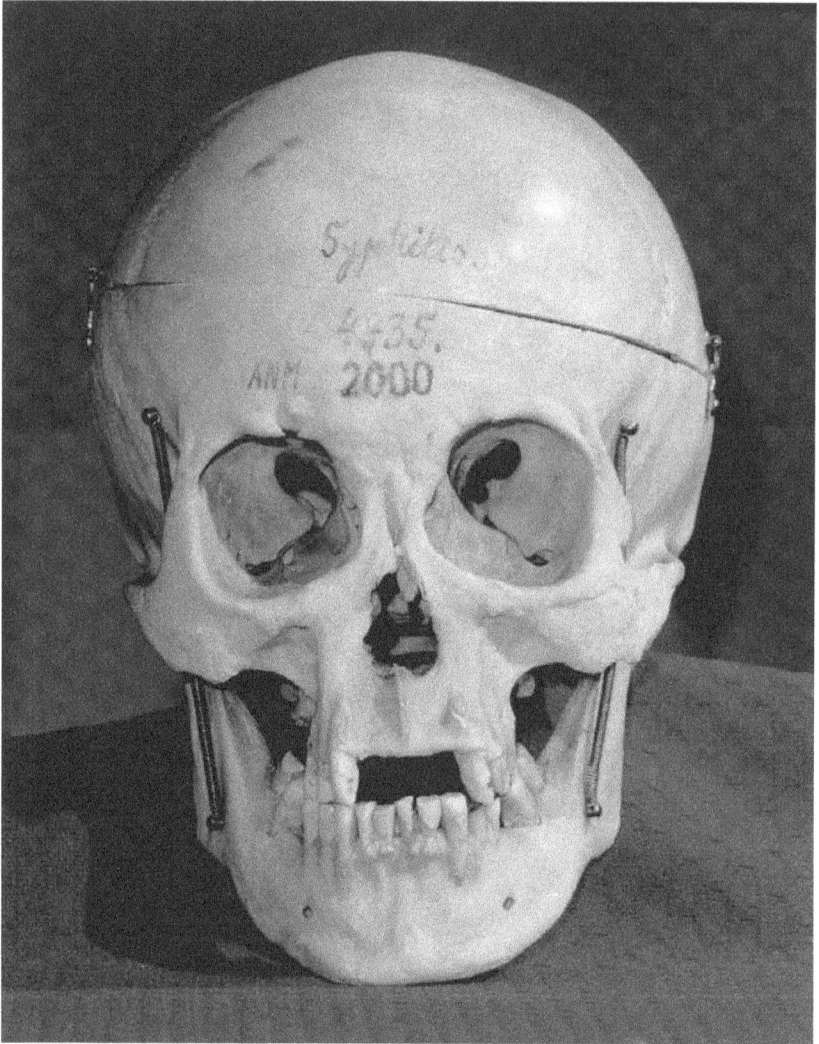

Figure 12. Facial skeleton destruction from growth alterations associated with congenital syphilis. (From Donald J. Ortner, image 001-470; used with his permission).

Another frequent alteration is the nasal passage, where many of the those thin bones are resorbed and even destroyed (Fig. 12). The most common syphilitic skeletal lesions, however, are front-to-back bowing of the lower legs, a distortion called saber shins for the saber shape they form (Fig. 13). Less frequent than the previous manifesta-

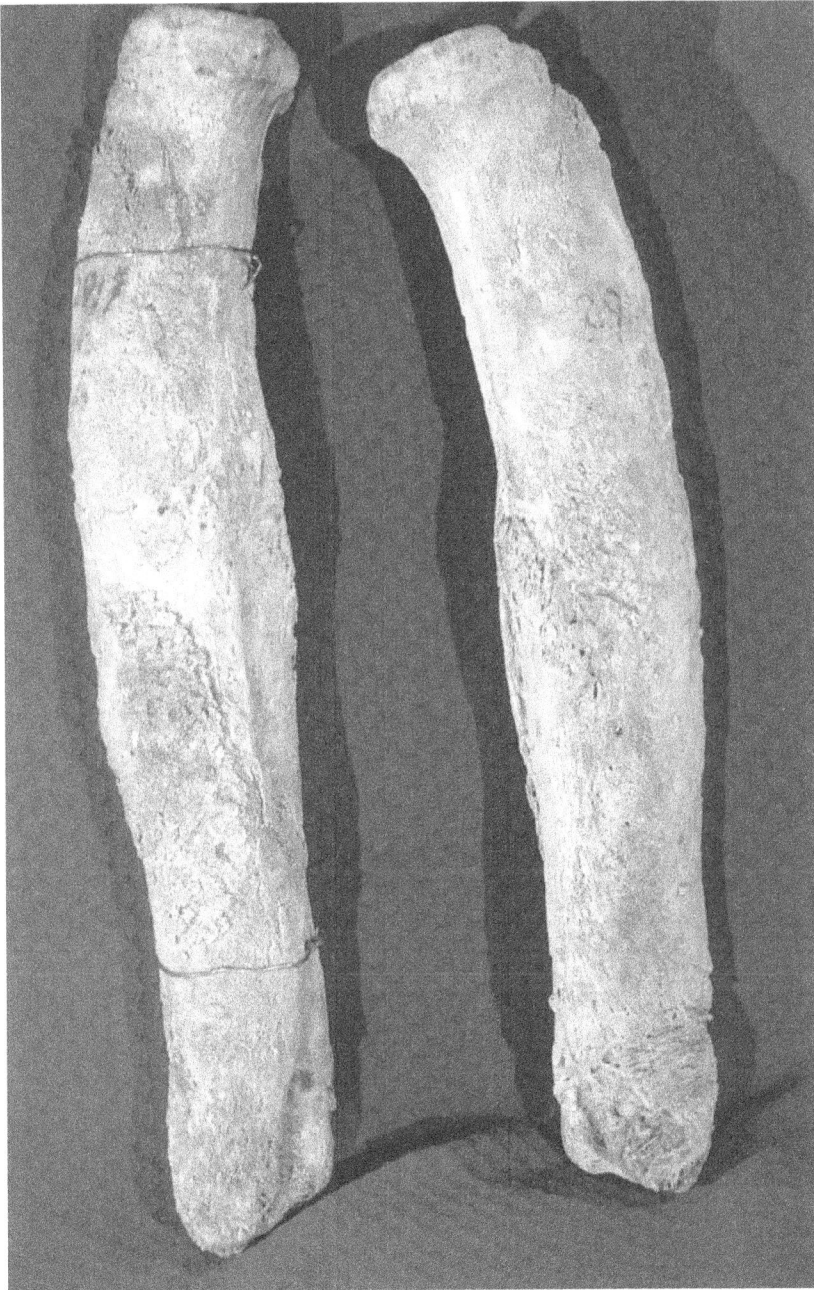

Figure 13. Tibia showing bowing ("saber shin") associated with tertiary syphilis. (From Donald J. Ortner, image 002-064; used with his permission).

tions, Charcot's joints (progressive deterioration of joints, especially knees) and gummatous lesions (localized soft, spongy defects) are also indicative of acquired syphilis. The three most common skeletal lesions (saber shins, cranial vault caries sicca and nasal passage destruction, in decreasing frequency) account for about 70% of the skeletal lesions (Ortner 2003:279). These most frequent manifestations of acquired venereal syphilis, then, are the ones most likely expected among the early 19th century adult Arikara skeletons. There is another suite of manifestations that the spirochete causes that needs to be considered before examining the Arikara skeletons.

As if the skeletal lesions of acquired venereal syphilis were not terrible enough, venereal syphilis may be visited upon the subsequent generation, transmitted to the fetus across the placental boundary. If the fetus survives the infection (recall that there is a 50% mortality rate among infected fetuses), post-uterine skeletal alterations may occur. The most diagnostic skeletal changes associated with congenital syphilis involve the facial elements and teeth. Growth-related malformations result in occlusally notched and screwdriver-shaped front teeth (Hutchinson's incisors) as well as misshapen molar crowns (Moon's molars) and malformed molar cusps (Fournier or mulberry molars). The facial skeleton may grow into a "saddle-shape" due to nasal area collapse (Fig. 12) and palatal loss. In addition, saber shins and generalized periostitis are common among those afflicted with congenital syphilis. More mature fetuses, full-term victims, and other young survivors may show other skeletal alterations, but they are often nondiagnostic as having been caused by syphilis and may have been caused by other agents (Ortner 2003: 289-297; Aufderheife and Rodriguez-Martin 1998:406, 595-596).

Summary

It is obvious that frequent promiscuous sex has ramifications. Accounts from the Lewis and Clark Expedition testify that there were venereal disease symptoms expressed by expedition members. These conclusions were supported by other observerers from the same period. There were standard treatments and based on the supplies the expedition took, they expected such eventualities. Syphilis seems to be the most likely disease based on timing and descriptions in the historic accounts. Although not all long-term sufferers of acquired or congenital syphilis display skeletal stigmata, those individuals who do may be diagnosed as having syphilis with some certainty—at least when other causes are excluded.

If the Arikara were harborers of venereal disease, as Lewis and Clark and some other early observers claim, then their skeletons should manifest the effects of these diseases. We are fortunate in this matter, at least in an empirical sense. There are a large number of skeletons from the Arikara villages that Lewis and Clark, Trudeau, Tabeau, Brackenridge, and Bradbury visited.

5. The Bones That Didn't Speak

The place where the Lewis and Clark Expedition met the Arikara in 1804 and 1806 was three villages. Those three villages were said to be the vestiges of 30-40 villages, earlier devastated by both epidemic diseases and warfare with the Teton Dakota. Many of those villages had their own social organization and political structure, including their own chiefs. By the time of the expedition's visits, the Arikara had been reduced to 2,000 souls, diminished from perhaps as many as 30,000 in the 18th century (Holder 1970:27).

Down but not out, the Arikaras had been decimated, but they were still a force to be reckoned with. The villages served as the center of Arikara social life and more broadly they were a pivotal trade center in a continent-wide aboriginal exchange network. Because of this pivotal position, twentieth century archaeologists, just as prehistoric traders and historic travelers, were drawn to the sites. Archaeologists recognized the importance the sites had for resolving many questions related to Arikara, including those concerning Arikara history and culture change, and that attention included Arikara skeletons. For our purposes, those skeletons prove critical for evaluating the historic accounts of venereal disease among the Arikara.

Before proceeding to the Arikara skeletons, we describe the Arikara villages, including their pivotal role in trade networks. Then we discuss the archaeology of the Arikara sites and their skeletons.

Arikara Villages and Lodges

The three Arikara villages Lewis and Clark visited were located a few miles up the Missouri River from the mouth of the Grand River. The location is now northern South Dakota, close to the North Dakota border (Fig. 2)—and not far from the hometown of Lawrence Welk, the maker of champagne music. As Krause (1972: 20) noted, the villages' location was geographically favorable for several reasons. St. Louis traders and trappers, who were headed to the fur-rich Northwest Plains, traveled by river to the Arikara villages, where they either traded for horses and went overland along the Grand River toward the Yellowstone River, or traded with the Arikara before continuing up the Missouri River. Similar advantages of the location extended into prehistory as indicated by the numerous, large prehistoric village sites found in the area.

In 1804, the three Arikara villages consisted of one on an island in the Missouri River (modern Ashley Island) and two villages on the west bank of the river about four miles above the island village (Fig. 2). The island village was abandoned by 1811, its residents apparently joining the west bank villages.

The west bank villages were located on grass-covered flats (Fig. 14). The edges of the flats were marked on the south by the Missouri River (which flows east-to-west here) and limited by low hills to the north. An intermittent stream, variously shown on maps as Cottonwood or Elk Creek, separated the two villages.

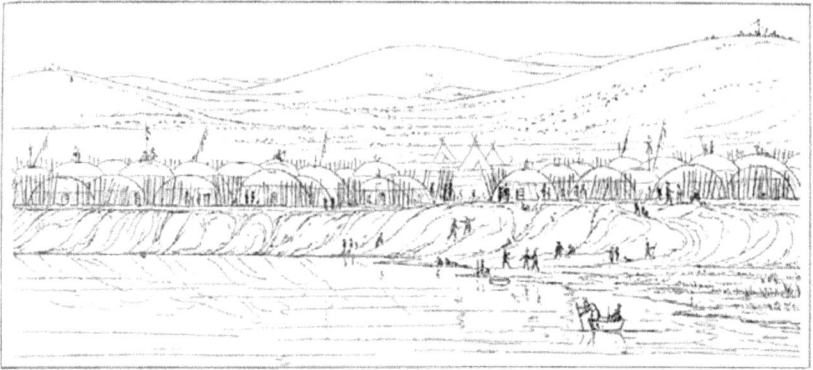

Riccaree village.

Figure 14. Catlin's (1926:229, fig. 80) drawing of the bank villages where Lewis and Clark visited the Arikara and where skeletons were excavated.

The villages were typical of late prehistoric Arikara communities. Each village consisted of 60 to 80 densely placed earth lodges, encircled by a dry moat with a log stockade inside the ditch (Krause 1972:16). An enemy foolish enough to attack the village faced a formidable fortification as well as a formidable adversary.

Protected by the fortification, earth lodges were the bee hives of Arikara life. The lodges were built by the industrious Arikara women and served as an extended family's home, ruled by an older woman. The Arikara earth lodge was shaped like an Eskimo's (Inuit's) igloo. As igloos, the earth lodges had a round footprint with a rectangular entrance hall.

Earth lodges were typically 30-50 feet in diameter, with a saucer-shaped floor dug several feet into the sod. The lodge superstructure was balanced on four posts set in holes near the center of the lodge with beams set on top of the posts forming a square. Long leaners ran from the lodge's pit edge toward the center, either over the top of an outside ring of posts-and-beams then on toward the lodge center or directly toward the lodge's center square. These structural members were covered with willows, twigs and grasses, then those covered with earth and sod. The earth insulated the lodges, making them cool during the summer's heat and efficiently heated in the winter by a centrally located hearth.

As efficient and comfortable as the lodges were in that harsh Northern Plains climate, they were not without their detractors. Tabeau's (Abel 1939:146) negative assessment of Arikara lodges went "an honest man has enough trouble to undergo there [trading with the Arikara] without depriving himself also of the sight of the sun, burying himself alive, and wallowing in the dirt. These lodges should be inhabited only by Ricaras, dogs, and bears."

At the lodge's top center was a hole for smoke to exit, with a central fire pit directly below the hole. In addition to the fire pit, cache pits, which were often bell-shaped in profile, were dug into the lodge floors and held the lauder from the gardens.

The Arikara's economy was based on maize horticulture supplemented with hunting, gathering and trading. The area around the villages supported several of those vocations. The Missouri River floodplain had tillable soil for their all-important gardens. There, in addition to corn, they grew beans and squash, supplemented by tobacco and other garden produce. The floodplain also had stands of cottonwood and willows, primary construction materials for lodges, stockades, other structures, as well as firewood. The grassy plains served as forage for the Arikara's horse herd, and the nearby prairie was periodically filled with game, most notably bison but including smaller game animals such as antelope. Spread across these ecological zones were wild plants—such as chokecherries, prairie turnips, cactus fruits, and grapes—that provided dietary variety and vitamins.

The Arikara food sources, although varied and usually more than sufficient for their dietary needs, were sometimes depleted. Late frosts, droughts and floods occasionally devastated crops. The bison herds sometimes wandered far from the villages. And wild plants produced only seasonally and some years produced poorly even when in season. When an alignment of these devastating events occurred, famine resulted. Some of the vicissitudes of planting, foraging and hunting were mitigated, however, by trading and bartering.

Arikara and the Aboriginal Trade Network

The Arikara villages occupied a strategic place for trading and the importance of trade must be underscored. Trade began long before the EuroAmerican traders arrived on the Upper Missouri River—or even the shores of America, for that matter. Prehistoric trade involved the Arikara and their neighbors as well as far-flung Native American groups. Precontact North America, in Wood's (1980:99) words, was "blanketed by a network of trails and trading relationships linking, to a greater or lesser degree, every tribe to one or more of its neighbors." Through this distribution system, materials from the Pacific Ocean and Gulf Coast found their way into Arikara hands long before the first European introduced himself. As an example, one author (TL) found a coral bead in an ant hill in northern New Mexico.

The Arikara were an important part of this prehistoric continent-wide network. In addition to their favorable geographic location, they occupied a permanent trading spot. They usually had a garden surplus. They conducted annual trade fairs. They provided means for peaceful gatherings. And they specialized in garden production. We consider each of these elements in turn.

Location, location, location is not only the realtors' mantra; it is the merchants' as well. A great shop in the wrong location leads the owner to financial ruin. The Arikara faced no such problem, at least not until later in the 19th century. They lived between two powerful trade spheres (Ewers 1968:14-33). To their south and west, there were the Cheyenne, Arapaho, Comanche, Kiowa Apache and Kiowa (Fig. 1), and through them in historic times they had access to

Spanish goods, including Spanish horses. To the east and south, their obstinate neighbors were the Teton Dakota, and through the Teton they had indirect contact with the other Dakotas and the annual rendezvous those tribes conducted (Fig. 1). All of these other tribes were nomadic and were hungry for what the Arikara had. It is as if the Arikara's village position was comparable to a mall location adjacent to the food court.

The Arikara's gardens and the hardworking Arikara women often produced a horticultural surplus. Their gardens were founded on the American vegetable tripod: corn, beans and squash, but included other garden produce, such as tobacco. The Arikara garden surplus was comparable to the modern home gardeners' late summer deluge of zucchinis and tomatoes. There was so much in a typical season, they could not give it all away.

Today's home gardeners rid themselves of their late summer surplus by foisting spare zucchinis and tomatoes on family and friends. The Arikara had a similar strategy. Their garden produce peaked in late summer, and their annual trade fair with the nomadic tribes coincided with this horticultural glut. Had Lewis and Clark arrived a month or two earlier than October, arriving in August or September 1804, they would have observed such a trade fair. These trade fairs were the Arikara's county fairs, but with much more. They involved gambling, fornicating, racing, gossiping, marrying and infecting—as well as trading (Wood 1980:106-107). As marriages, fairs work well when the participants are getting along, but poorly between warring factions, as these tribes often were.

Fairs involving hostile groups required a plan—a truce, if not a peace, for the duration of the event. The Arikara had a solution, what might be called "pax Arikara" or what Wood (1980:104) termed "market peace." Here was how it worked. While within sight of the Arikara villages, animosities were to be set aside. So the dastardly

Teton, for example, who may have killed several Arikara the previous week, would have free passage into and around the Arikara villages during the trade fair. This protection persisted as long as they stayed. But once they left sight of the villages, old animosities and vengeances reappeared and hostilities recommenced. These peaceful interludes for the trade fairs lasted no longer than a modern Mideast peace accord.

In addition to peaceful interactions, these trade relationships also required groups to intensify their exploitation and production in somewhat specialized spheres. The Arikara produced an agricultural surplus, and the nomads produced a surplus from hunting and gathering. Nevertheless either group, at least potentially, could have produced anything the other groups had. For instance, the semi-sedentary Arikara could—and did—hunt as well as garden. Some nomadic groups, such as the Cheyenne, had grown crops but decided to follow game and emphasize hunting. The nomad trading partners, for their part in the deal, brought meats, furs and handicrafts (Wood 1980:100). These specializations extended from the prehistoric past into the historic period, what Ewers (in Wood 1980:103) dubbed an "elaboration of a prehistoric trade pattern."

To conclude this discussion of trade, there are several important points. Trade caused cultural diffusion. Goods and ideas, people and diseases spread rapidly through these trade networks, and in historic times with the addition of horses, distances traveled expanded and speed of travel increased (Wood 1980:106). Although Wood was referring primarily to the notorious epidemic diseases, such as smallpox and measles, the same trade networks enhanced the dissemination of venereal diseases from one tribe to the next.

Finally, the Arikara's affluence and prime trading location, profitable as it was, proved to be their undoing (Wood 1980:106). When the white traders entered the Arikara trade network, they found ready customers and a tradition of trading. The difference from prehistoric trade was that the white man's trade goods were made with materials and techniques unavailable to the Indians. What white merchant would trade a mirror for ten pumpkins? He had no need for so many pumpkins. A bullet-casting mold outbid vast quantities of dried bison jerky. Worse still for the Arikaras, the white traders began to barter directly with the horse nomads, cutting out the Arikara middleman, and whites later moved upstream, intercepting other potential Arikara customers and becoming trappers themselves.

Initial relations between the Arikara and white travelers during the 18th and early 19th centuries were warm. But as mentioned in more detail in a previous chapter, in 1823, open hostilities erupted between the Arikara villagers and Ashley's traders, resulting in the deaths of a dozen traders. Col. Henry Leavenworth retaliated with a punitive campaign against the Arikara, his forces including his regiment, supplemented by traders, traders and Ashley's employees as well as several hundred Dakota warriors. They surrounded the two Arikara bank villages, but after a few days of negotiating and skirmishing, the Arikara escaped during the dark of night, leaving the villages to Leavenworth's forces. The Arikara abandoned the villages for a year, some living in the north near the Mandan, and others in the south with the Pawnee. They reoccupied the bank villages by 1825, where they remained until 1832, when the villages were permanently abandoned (Krause 1972:15).

These villages were the last location where the Arikara led a relatively autonomous life. After abandoning the villages and following a few years of wandering, the Arikara settled close to the horticultural Mandan and Hidatsa in North Dakota, as Lewis and Clark had counseled them to do a few decades earlier. The tribes united to become the Three Affiliated Tribes, now living on Ft. Berthold

Indian Reservation in western North Dakota. But that was far in the future when Lewis and Clark visited.

Leavenworth Site and Its Skeletons

The 19th century Arikara site attracted the attention of many 20th century archaeologists. Dubbed the Leavenworth Site, alternatively known as the Lewis and Clark Site, it includes the two Arikara bank villages (Fig. 15). The third village, the one on an island about 4 miles downstream from the bank villages, was apparently destroyed in the early 19th century by changes in the Missouri River.

The Arikara bank villages were excavated by archaeologists in the 1900s before the site was inundated by the Corps of Engineers' Oahe Reservoir in the 1960s. Located on the bluffs above and about 200 yards north of the villages, the Leavenworth Site cemeteries were excavated by William H. Over of the University of South Dakota in the 1910s, Mathew W. Stirling and William Duncan Strong of the Smithsonian Institution's National Museum of Natural History in the 1920s and 1930s (Wedel 1955), and William M. Bass, then of the University of Kansas, in the 1960s (Fig. 16). With the exception of Bass, these archaeologists also excavated portions of the villages. Richard Krause, then of the University of Missouri, with University of Nebraska field schools in 1960 and 1961 as well as two shorter periods, excavated other portions of the villages (Krause 1972:22).

Altogether these archaeologists recovered more than 300 skeletons from the site (Table 1). There were also two skeletons excavated by Preston Holder of the University of Nebraska in 1962, but those apparently were from an earlier cultural component, one predating the historic Arikara occupation by more than 100 years (Extended Coalescent Period, AD 1550-1675; http://www.cr.nps.gov/nagpra/fed_notices/nagpradir/nic0656.html; NAGPRA Notice dated October 10, 2002, accessed June 28, 2006). Those two skeletons

Table 1. Skeletal remains excavated from Leavenworth Site (from Bass et al. 1971:18, table 1).

Archaeologists	Institutional Affiliation	Excavation Years	Number of Skeletons	Major Publications
William H. Over	University of South Dakota	1915, 1917	15	
Matthew W. Stirling	Smithsonian Institution	1923	33	Stirling 1924; Wedel 1955
William Duncan Strong	Smithsonian Institution	1932	4	Strong 1940; Wedel 1955
William M. Bass	Kansas University	1965, 1966	285	Bass et al. 1971; Shermis 1969

are not of interest to us and excluded from further consideration here.

If the historic accounts, including those of Lewis and Clark, accurately depict the presence of venereal disease among the historic Arikara, then some of the Leavenworth Site skeletons should display the osseous indications of those diseases. Most definitively, acquired syphilis should be indicated by caries sicca and saber shins; congenital syphilis by Hutchinson's incisors, nasal-palatal growth alterations and changes in the lower leg bones; and gonorrhea by arthritis of the knees and ankles. There are other generalized, nonspecific indicators of infections that may have been caused by venereal diseases, although these manifestations are less diagnostic than those just mentioned. So, what do the bones say? Do they show signs of venereal disease?

Stirling and Strong recovered 37 skeletons that were—and perhaps still are—at the Smithsonian Institution. They, along with all of the other skeletons attributed to the Arikara, have undergone analysis by the Smithsonian Institution's Repatriation Office in preparation for delivery to the Three Affiliated Tribes of North Dakota.

THE LEAVENWORTH SITE, 39C09
Corson County

Map drawn by Maurice E. Kirby

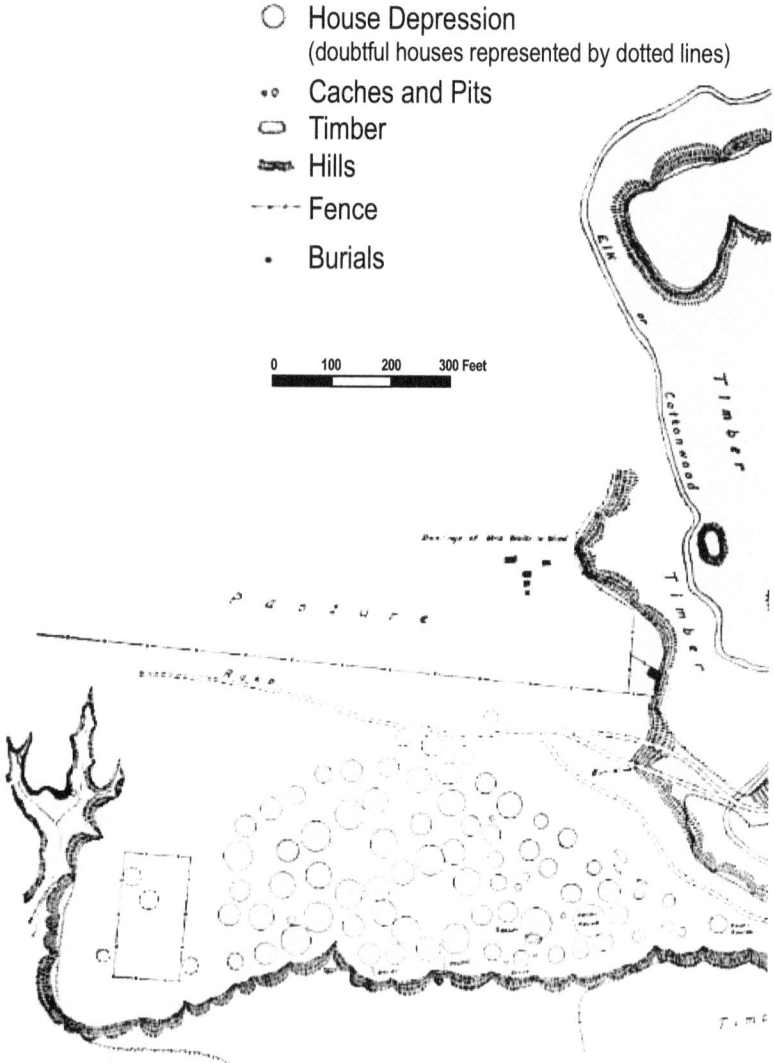

N

○ **House Depression**
(doubtful houses represented by dotted lines)

•○ **Caches and Pits**

▭ **Timber**

Hills

---·· **Fence**

• **Burials**

0   100   200   300 Feet

Figure 15. Maurice Kirby's map of the Leavenworth Site showing lodges and burials on hills to north. (Modiied from Bass et al. 1971:17, fig. 4; used with permission of University of Kansas Anthropology Department).

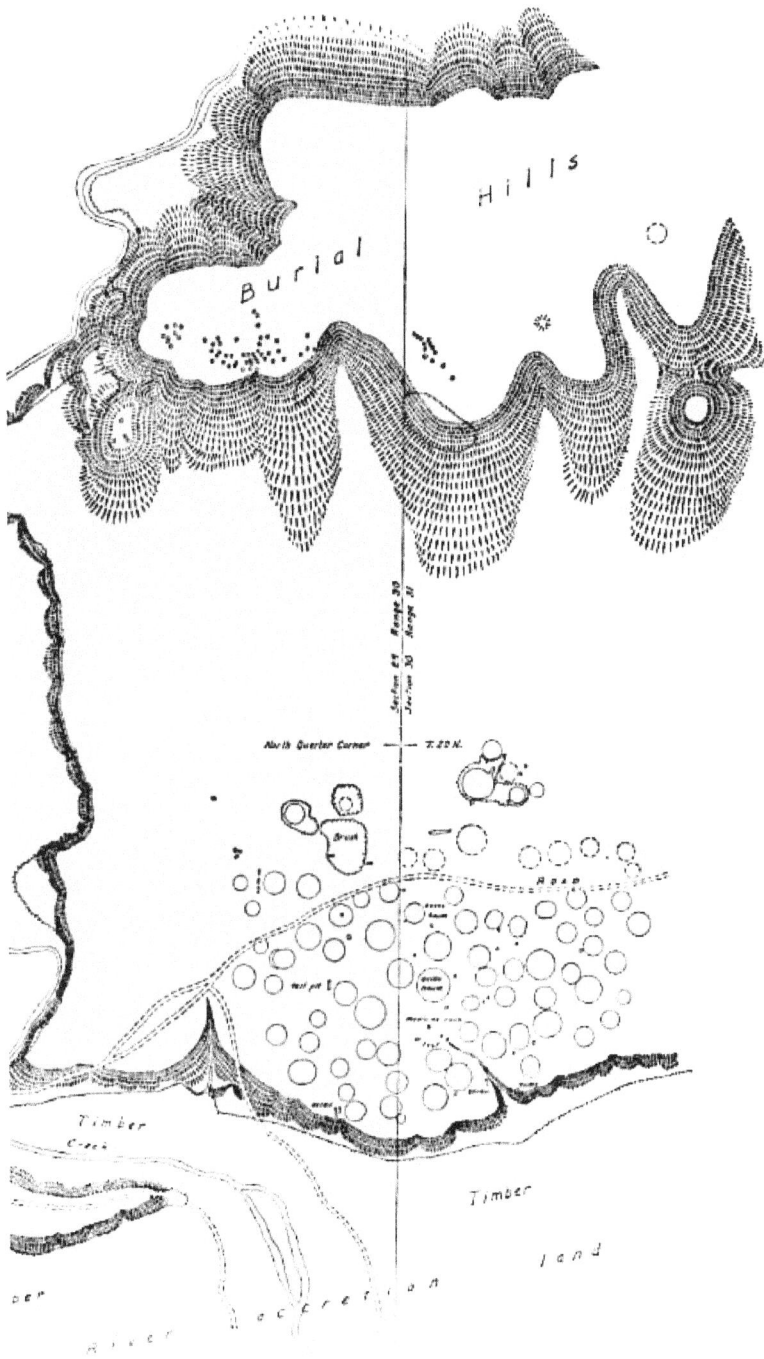

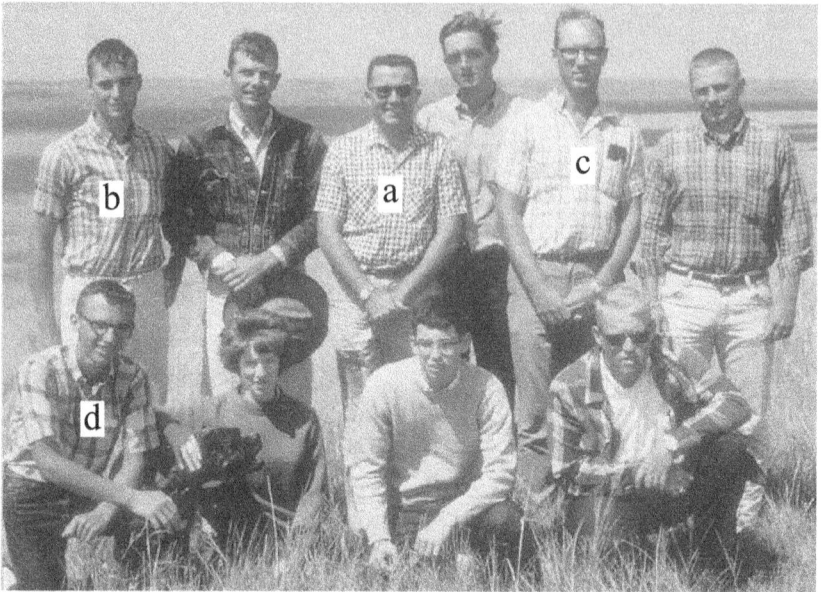

Figure 16. University of Kansas archaeologists of the Leavenworth Site, summer 1965. a. William M. Bass, project director and senior author of Leavenworth skeleton monograph, b. Douglas H. Ubelaker, excavator who wrote senior honors thesis on Leavenworth teeth, c. Richard L. Jantz, crew chief, co-author of Leavenworth monograph and long-term Arikara researcher, and d. P. Willey, excavator and co-author of this work. Other persons shown are so famous they need no introductions. (Used with kind permission of W.M. Bass)

William H. Over's material is further along the repatriation process. After being examined by Owsley and co-workers (Owsley and Jantz 1994) as well as the Greggs (1987), the Over Leavenworth Site skeletons were repatriated by the State of South Dakota and reburied in the 1980s (Jim Haug, personal communication November 10, 2006).

The Leavenworth Cemetery skeletons that Bass (Fig. 16) excavated are both the largest sample from the site, and they are the most thoroughly reported. Bass et al. (1971) published a lengthy monograph, Ubelaker (1971) described the dentitions as an appendix in Bass's monograph, Shermis (1969) reported the skeletons' paleopathology as his MA thesis, and the Greggs (1987) included some of these materials in their paleopathology summary of "Dakota Territory" skeletons.

Shermis's study of Bass's Leavenworth skeletons is the most likely of the publications to identify lesions associated with venereal disease. He examined the skeletons for many different kinds of diseases. He found few neoplasms ("cancers"), most likely infrequent due to the youthful age of the skeletons. He believed that there were some nutritional defects, indicating periods of starvation. He found frequent fractures and both arrow and bullet wounds, which he attributed to warfare, "dangerous games," and domestic violence—an issue he elaborated in a later publication (Shermis 1982-84). Most importantly for our purposes, he described infections, and presumably including the treponemal infections—had they been present.

He dedicated a chapter to the infectious diseases, as well as noting infections as alternative diagnoses of other diseases in other chapters. Approximately 10% of the individuals Shermis (1969:38) reported had one or more inflammatory lesions. He identified 28 individuals with a total of 47 bones displaying infectious lesions. There were inflammatory lesions from the youngest age group through the oldest. The young tended to have ear infections. The adults, in addition to those lesions, had other infections involving the trunk and limb skeletons. Some of the alterations were superficial, others were penetrating and deep.

Among these infections, there was no mention of any of the classic indicators of acquired syphilis. There was no caries sicca and no saber shins. In addition, there was no mention of the growth alterations associated with congenital syphilis. There was no saddle-shaped or collapsed nasal area. As Shermis's work, the Greggs' (1987) compendium of Middle Missouri River skeletal pathologies does not mention any treponemal diseases from the Leavenworth Site.

Ubelaker analyzed the dental materials of the same Leavenworth skeletons that Bass et al. described and Shermis reported. Among other observations, Ubelaker (1971:184-186) examined anterior teeth for crown variations, such as shovel- and peg-shaped incisors, but made no note of the even-more striking Hutchinson's incisors associated with congenital syphilis. He examined the molars for cusp pattern, extra cusps, impaction, but reported no Moon's or mulberry molars that are associated with congenital syphilis (Ubelaker 1971: 188-192). He also described dental pathologies, including carious lesions, abscesses, antemortem tooth loss, calculus, and even previously unreported interproximal grooves (Ubelaker 1971:192-193), but made no note of the dental stigmata associated with congenital syphilis. Based on this absence of such dental traits in Ubelaker's appendix and lack of diagnostic skeletal lesions in Shermis's thesis, we conclude that there were no dental or skeletal indicators of congenital syphilis among the Arikara Leavenworth Site skeletons.

In summary, there is no evidence of venereal syphilis among the early 19th Arikara skeletons from the Leavenworth Site. Not only are there no instances at the Leavenworth Site, there have been few, if any, substantiated cases reported from the Northern Plains.

Syphilis on the Plains?

There is a recent summary of the syphilis-like skeletal diseases reported from the prehistoric Plains (Hodges and Schermer 2005) as well as an older classic assessment (Gregg and Gregg 1987). These syphilis-like diseases, it should be noted, could be other diseases, most likely the other treponemal diseases. The other two treponemal diseases that cause bone changes are bejel and yaws. The former is found today in the Middle East, while the latter is a tropical disease. Neither seems likely in the Upper Missouri River Basin region, but neither has been discussed extensively by researchers.

Based on the published syntheses, we summarize the skeletal evidence for syphilis chronologically by archaeological periods, beginning with the earliest. Although there have been no claims of such manifestations among the earliest PaleoIndian Period (9,000 years ago and older), perhaps due to small sample sizes, the next period has the best substantiated claim of syphilitic manifestations.

The earliest and also the most likely case of venereal syphilis on the Plains is from the Archaic Period. The Archaic Period people's economy was based on foraging and hunting. The site of interest (ca. 2500 years BP) in Saskatchewan (Walker 1983) had a skeleton with what appears to have been a syphilis-induced aortic aneurysm. Bones adjacent to the aorta remodeled, demonstrating the plastic qualities of both the artery and bones. The posterior surface of the manubrium, medial end of the right clavicle and left bodies of thoracic vertebrae 2 and 3 showed cavitations. In conclusion, the skeletal modifications were consistent with tertiary syphilis involving the cardiovascular system and secondarily affecting adjacent bone surfaces. The specimen shows relatively certain evidence of syphilis, but is from a site that was occupied more than 2300 years before occupation of Leavenworth Site and more than 500 miles from that Arikara site.

Following that period, the Plains Woodland Period continued the foraging and hunting of the previous Archaic Period, supplemented with some horticulture involving corn, beans and squash. Pottery- and burial mound-making also occurred. Several Woodland Period burial mounds (Swift Bird, Grover Hand and Arpan sites) are located 30 miles downstream from the Leavenworth Site. They dated ca. AD 100-400. Many of these Woodland skeletons, from sites located a few miles away, have lesions of the lower legs that may be attributed to treponemal diseases. However it is unclear which treponemal disease or diseases were involved (Bass and Phenice 1975).

More recent than the Woodland Period is the Villager Period. It was a time of larger, more permanent settlements, with greater reliance on horticultural products for subsistence than the previous periods. In the late prehistoric, there are several sites with skeletons that have been identified with treponemal manifestations. Some are indicated from Middle Missouri Tradition individuals at Site 39CA102, and others at Crow Creek Site (Coalescent Tradition, ca. AD 1350), where at least 486 individuals were murdered and their skeletons buried in a dry moat surrounding the village. Violence was not the only problem at Crow Creek. Saber shins were reported there as well as 39CA102.

Later in the Villager Period than the two sites just mentioned, is the protohistoric Mobridge Site (ca AD 1750). Located near the mouth of the Grand River, a few miles downstream from the Leavenworth Site, many of the Mobridge Site skeletons have periosteal swellings and gummatous lesions, primarily on the tibiae and fibulae, suggesting treponeal disease, although the analyst did not specify which one or ones were present (Palkovich 1981).

From the Historic Period (most likely 1880s), a Sioux child from central South Dakota has what appears to be Hutchinson's incisors—the dental malformation due to congenital syphilis. The trait may have been misdiagnosed by the original authors (Willey and Swegle 1980). This specimen post-dates the Arikara Leavenworth Site by 50 years and the skeleton is attributed to the Dakota, who alternated between being the trading partners and enemies of the Arikara.

There are two other Plains skeletal specimens that have distinctive lesions but whose proveniences are questionable or unknown. One South Dakota skeleton displays a possible Charcot joint (Gregg and Gregg 1987:62) and there are possible Hutchinson's incisors from a North Dakota site (Williams cited in Gregg and Gregg 1987: 62). Without precise provenience, however, no definitive inferences can be made from these observations concerning syphilis among the Northern Plains Natives.

In summary, there are some Great Plains skeletons that have disease alterations that may be venereal syphilis. Treponeal disease, more broadly, has been identified from the Missouri River region in periods before and decades after the Leavenworth Site occupation. Venereal syphilis is only one of the four treponemal diseases, however; the other treponemal diseases have not been excluded in most of these diagnoses. And there seems to be only one probable early case of syphilis on the Plains. So, if venereal syphilis was endemic on the Plains, either in prehistoric or historic times, there is little tangible skeletal evidence of its presence.

6. Historic and Ethnographic Explanations

The absence of skeletal lesions indicating syphilis among the historic Leavenworth Site Arikara bones contradicts the historic accounts. If the historic accounts are accurate, then some of the Leavenworth Site skeletons should have syphilitic lesions, but that is not the case. There are many possible explanations for the absence of skeletal manifestations of syphilis among the Arikara skeletons from the Leavenworth Site. We present those explanations in two broad categories: one involving historic and ethnographic evidence presented in this chapter, and the other involving skeletal and biological data presented in the next chapter.

We explore several historic and ethnographic explanations. The first possibility is that the historic chroniclers misdiagnosed or misrepresented the diseases that their party members experienced. If, on the other hand, the observers correctly identified the diseases, there are two alternate explanations. It is possible that the Arikara had effective medical treatments for the diseases, thus curing or at least diminishing the effects of the illnesses so that the diseases were thwarted and their skeletal alterations eliminated or at least diminished. A final explanation is that the Arikara had special mortuary treatment of the afflicted that precluded archaeological recovery for the syphilitic skeletons. Each explanation is considered in turn.

Erroneous Historic Diagnoses

The first explanation calls into question the veracity—or at least the accuracy—of the historic accounts. According to this explanation, the discrepancy between the historic accounts and skeletal lesions is explained by the chroniclers making erroneous claims and the Leavenworth Site skeletons accurately depicting the absence of syphilis among the Arikara. Is it possible that Lewis and Clark may have misdiagnosed the illness?

The Lewis and Clark Expedition visited Arikara in the early 1800s, a century before reliable diagnostic laboratory techniques were available to definitively identify the disease. Their visit, in fact, happened even before the germ theory of disease was accepted by Western medicine. What was the state of early 19th century medicine?

The two major venereal diseases recognized in the early 19th century—syphilis and gonorrhea—were identified as separate disease entities based on Benjamin Bell's 1793 distinctions of the two. Although the diseases were distinguished from one another, they were generally considered merely different expressions of the same disease (Chuinard 1979:265 fn, 312 fn). It was only later in the 19th century, after the germ theory of disease gained a foothold, that the two illnesses were distinguished as separate diseases cased by different microorganisms.

In 1879 Albert Neisser identified the gonococcus microbe as the cause of gonorrhea. The cause of syphilis, however, remained a mystery as late as 1892, when Osler wrote that the source was "a virus whose exact nature is unknown." Previously, the 1857 Webster's dictionary defined virus as "active or contagious matter." In brief, physicians had known for 500 years that it was spread by sexual contact, but the underlying biological mechanism defied the science then available. And only in 1905—a century after Lewis and Clark's Expedition— did Fritz Schaudinn identify the spirochete *Treponema pallidum* as the cause of syphilis.

So, Lewis and Clark, before the advent of germ theory and before definitive laboratory tests, would have diagnosed venereal disease from the most superficial and obvious signs and complaints: skin lesions and painful urination. Could they have misdiagnosed the disease or diseases involved?

It seems unlikely that such worldly observers as Lewis and Clark would be in error in this matter, at least on purpose. In addition to their previous military experience with ardent young men, Lewis received instruction concerning illnesses and medical treatments from Dr. Benjamin Rush in Philadelphia. A signatory of the Declaration of Independence, Rush was among the US's most eminent physicians of the day. And both captains had access to Dr. Antoine Francois Saugrain's advice while wintering near St. Louis in preparation for proceeding up the Missouri River and to the Pacific Ocean (Chuinard 1979:265). The captains' background, experience, and training must have included identification and treatment of venereal disease.

And even if Lewis and Clark were in error, it is unlikely so many other and independent observers would make the same error. Trudeau, Tabeau and Bradbury knew the Arikara from the same time period, and all made similar observations concerning venereal disease complaints. These ol' boys knew their venereal diseases!

Such broad-spread misrepresentation would only be possible if there was a concerted conspiratorial smear campaign against the Arikara. As preposterous as this claim seems, consider for a moment the following information. There was—and still is—prejudice involved with the sexual transmission of syphilis and there was a widespread 19th century perception of Native Americans being dissolute.

The perception of the Arikara women as the source of syphilis, for instance, is in keeping with the concepts of early 19th century syphilis (Gilman 1988:254-255). During the 18th century, syphilis transmission was perceived as coming from the "corrupt female," shifting the source of the disease from men, portraying men instead as the victims (Gilman 1988:254). By the early 19th century in particular, the concept of "seductress as source of pollution" was so well entrenched (Gilman 1988:256) that Jean-Louis Alibert's 1806 text on dermatology depicted all syphilitics as females, none as males (Gilman 1988:255). In addition to notions of syphilis-festering females, there is another aspect to these concepts involving Native Americans.

Disease, be it venereal or not, is often attributed to "others:" other groups and other places. Consider Asian avian flu as a recent example. In 19th century Western culture, syphilis was often associated with prostitutes—who were perceived as both socially fallen and sexually deviant, living outside normal polite society. It is a small step to extend this otherness from prostitutes to members of other cultures. Sexually available Native American women fit this mental template. The historic accounts of the Arikara smack of these prejudices—outsider seductresses (Arikara women) engaged in deviant behavior (extramarital sex trade) transmitting contagion to clients (Canadians, boatmen, Creoles and enlisted men), who themselves were on the periphery of Western mainstream. Concepts of illness and health can be used as tools of domination, just as gun powder and lead, and political and military subjugation.

This explanation that the 19th century observers were wrong, whether it was purposeful or inadvertent, seems unlikely. Syphilis was common in the 19th century. All observant travelers would have been familiar with its more common forms. Some travelers provided surprising insights and details, for instance Bradbury's account of "his" Canadians' illnesses and their remedies. There is also a general similarity among the observations, all recognizing and noting venereal disease among the Arikara. Taking all of these details together, this explanation of erroneous diagnosis is unlikely.

Ready Remedies

Some accounts suggest that the Arikara had medicines and understanding of cures for sexually transmitted —as well as many other—diseases. Centuries of illness exposure, sickness and healing brought forth cultural means to identify, explain and deal with illnesses. As modern medicine, some tribal remedies were effective and successful; others were ineffective.

If effective traditional cures for venereal diseases were known by the historic Arikara and those treatments were applied early in the course of syphilis, the progress of the disease might be halted, perhaps even a cure effected. In that case, no tertiary skeletal changes would occur, and the Leavenworth Site skeletons would not be affected. To understand the context of such healing, we present the Arikara doctors who conducted the healing, Arikara concepts of illness, and Arikara means of curing.

Doctors

Arikara doctors or "medicine men" had prestige. At times they were honored and at other times they were feared. Overall they held high status, second in rank only to the chiefs and priests of the leading Arikara families (Parks 2001:375).

In traditional Arikara society, there were two kinds of doctors (Fig. 17). The first kind of Arikara physician included individuals who had acquired special healing powers outside the established medical societies, usually power bestowed from a spirit directly to

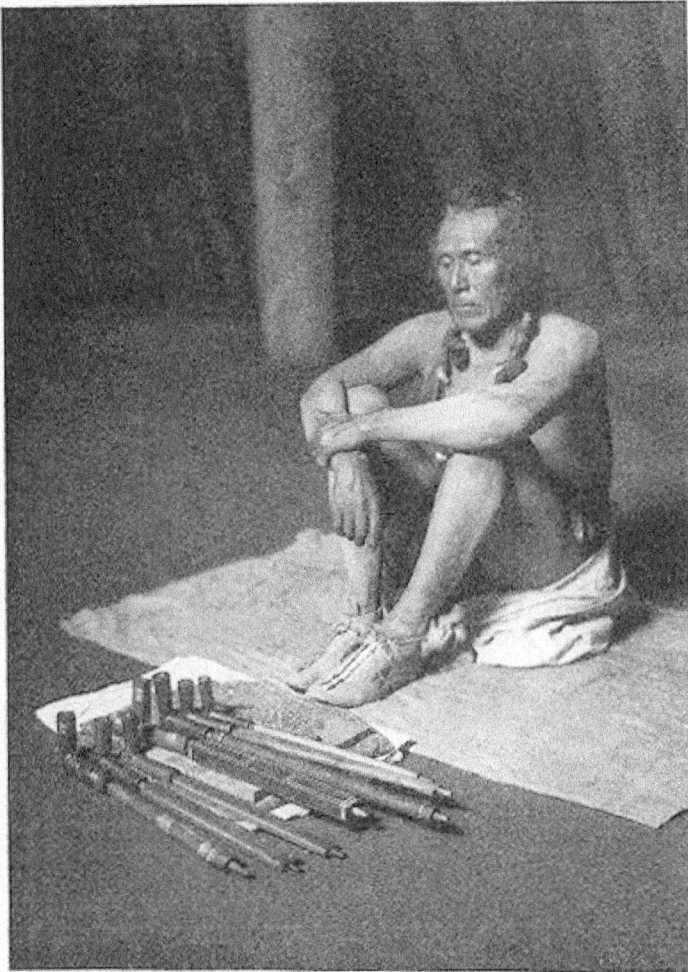

Figure 17. Edward Curtis's "In the Medicine Lodge," photographed in early 20th century (Used with permission of Northwestern University Library.)

that person (Parks 2001:381). As such, their rituals were more idiosyncratic and specific to the practioner, and their status in Arikara society was based largely on their individual charisma and healing successes.

The other kind of Arikara doctors became medicine men through initiation and achievement within established medical societies or fraternities, each of which possessed a medicine bundle. Even in the early 1900s, the Arikara still recognized nine such medical associations (Curtis 1907-1930, 5:64). Membership in these societies tended to be passed along family lines, aided by the family wealth that was required for initiation into medical associations and for purchasing knowledge to ascend through the organization's ranks.

The special knowledge that senior medicine men possessed was guarded and only passed to junior practioners with reluctance and at dear costs. Acquiring such knowledge was achieved in several ways. Most notably an initiate's wife could act as an intermediary, having sex with an established, knowledgeable doctor of the society, who passed the power and secrets from the established doctor to the wife. The wife, in turn, transmitted the power and secrets to her husband (Parks 2001:383). This transmission is similar to that previously mentioned concerning the expedition members. Following many such transmissions, the novice eventually gained considerable spiritual power and medical knowledge, and the more he possessed, the greater his standing within his medical society as well as within Arikara society more generally (Curtis 1907-1930:64).

In the traditional Arikara annual cycle, the medical societies held lengthy summer ceremonies that lasted two or three weeks. During that period, the doctors virtually lived in the medicine lodge, a special earth lodge, similar but larger than the usual habitation lodge. It was located near the center of the village (Parks 2001:381). When the Lewis and Clark Expedition visited the Arikara in 1804, the medicine society ceremonies had peaked two months before they arrived and were completed by the time of their visit. The most detailed descriptions of the medicine ceremonies were written 100 years after Lewis and Clark's Arikara visit. Edwin Curtis (1907-1930,

94

5:59-100) observed and photographed a reconstruction of some ceremonies, when they were staged for him following a 20-year hiatus in the ceremonies' performance.

Illness

Traditional Arikara believed that illness was caused by spirits that were sent by nefarious beings and by spells that were cast by antagonistic medicine men to make people sick or even to kill them. Many traditional societies have concepts of illnesses being caused by supernatural means. As Tabeau (Abel 1939:183) wrote concerning the Arikara's concepts of illness, "there prevails no natural sickness, as all illness is either the result of the vengeance of some angry spirit or a succession of evil deeds of a magician...." All societies have means of conceptualizing and dealing with such eventualities. Treatments and medicines are the ones we consider in the next sections

Cures

As would be expected if illnesses were produced by supernatural causes, the Arikara cures also invoked supernatural intervention. Tabeau (Abel 1939:183) noted that the Arikara doctors used songs to counteract the illness-causing evil spirits and sorcerers, sung while they rubbed patients with their hands and other objects. Following repetitious and lengthy performances, the "charlatans," as Tabeau dubbed them, concluded the ceremonies by sucking foreign objects from patients' bodies.

The Arikara perfected legerdemain and were unexcelled at this skill. Even the jaded Tabeau, who had little good to write about them, recognized the Arikara's supremacy in these skills. Before Tabeau's (Abel 1939:188) amazed eyes, a medicine man changed a leather garter into a "living adder" and back and forth ten times. One medicine man struck another with a hatchet, killing him, only to have the corpse brought back to life by a third doctor (Abel 1939:188). Tabeau

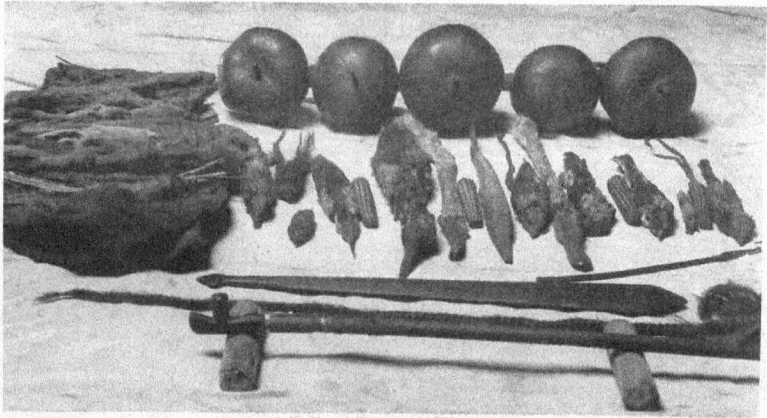

Figure 18. Edward Curtis's "Contents of Arikara Tribal Medicine Bundle" photographed in early 20th century. Note many plants as well as bird carcasses. (Used with permission of Northwestern University Library.)

(Abel 1939:188-189) told other stories of seeing men being shot, a knife piercing parts of the body, and an arrow drawn through a heart, all of which were healed before his very eyes. But magic tricks, as remarkable as they were, were only one part of curing the sick.

There is a detailed account of a healing ceremony provided by one of the early travelers. Barrister Brackenridge (1906:117), while walking through an Arikara village in 1811, observed the healing ceremony of a boy, who he described as having slight pleurisy. Brackenridge noted that the healing procedure began with rigorous massage of the boy. When that procedure failed to cure him, there were chants, dances and blowing on the patient. In addition to these physical manipulations and spiritual implorations, Brackenridge observed some plants that the Arikara doctor used in the medical procedures, plants that mainstream Western medicine might interpret as a treatment with pharmaceutical properties that could be empirically tested (Fig. 18).

96

Plants were frequently employed in traditional Arikara medicine. There are several sources of information concerning medicinal plants that the Arikara may have employed. We consider the sources starting with the broadest level and proceed to the narrowest spectrum.

The first source of information concerns plants that are available on the Great Plains and that were used by traditional Native American tribes other than the Arikara to treat venereal disease (Table 2). This approach provides a list of plants that the Arikara could have potentially employed to treat the sexually transmitted ailments that Lewis and Clark, and others described.

First a note about the sources used to establish this table is in order. The list is a compilation using several sources. First, the Great Plains Flora Association's (1986) *Flora of the Great Plains* was consulted as well as James Duke's (2002) *Handbook of Medicinal Herbs*. The plants in Duke's venereal disorders section that were also in the flora list were noted (courtesy of Jim Bauml). Also examined was the University of Michigan's list of herbs (http://herb.umd.umich.edu/herb/search.pl, accessed June 22, 2006).

This hodge-podge of plants used to treat venereal diseases (Table 2) provides a broad perspective to plants used by Native Americans as well as in Colonial America. On the face of it, the list appears lengthy and useful, but closer inspection displays holes and tatters. Many of the plants do not grow in the Dakotas and would have had to be transported long distances to reach Arikara hands. Examples include *Actaea pachypoda*, *Ephedra nevadensis*, *Hydrangea arboresncens*, and others. In addition to distance from the Arikara, other plants were introduced from outside the continent and probably not available to the Arikara until after Lewis and Clark's visit. Those plants include *Arctium lappa*, *Rumex crispus*, and many others.

Table 2. Plants used by Native Americans to treat venereal diseases, (From Great Plains Flora Association's *Flora of the Great Plains*, 1986, and James Duke's *CRC Handbook of Medicinal Herbs*, 2002 courtesy of Jim Bauml, except as noted in Source column. Information also from http://herb.umd.umich.edu/herb/search.pl, accessed June 22, 2006).

Scientific Name	Common Name	Tribe	Medical Summary	Source
Actaea pachypoda	White baneberry		[Plant not collected or documented in Dakotas]	
Apocynum	Dogbane	Chickasaw & Choctaw	*A. cannabinum* (Indian hemp) –syphilis. Kindscher, p. 43.	
Arctostaphylos uva-ursi	Kinnikinnick			
Arctium lappa	Greater burdock		[Introduced plant]	
Asclepias syriaca	Common milkweed			
Caulophyllum thalictroides	Blue cohosh			
Ephedra nevadensis	Nevada jointfir		[Restricted to W & SW US; not documented or collected in Dakotas] Venereal disease, Martinez‡	
Equisetum arvense	Field horsetail	Mesquakies	*E. hyemale* – gonorrhea. Kindscher, p. 241	
Eupatorium perfoliatum	Common boneset		Treat gonorrhea; Kindscher p. 105, citing Shemluck 1982. Not collected in Dakotas.	
Grindelia squarrosa	Curlycup gumweed	Gros Ventres & Shoshone	Tea for VD (Crees treated gonorrhea). Kindscher, p. 120	
Hydrangea arborescens	Wild hydrangea		[Not collected or documented in Dakotas; only Eastern & more Southern states]	
Juniperus communis*	Common juniper	Blackfoot	Berry decoction used to treat VDs	Hart 1992: 37; Johnston 1987:17
Liatris "pycnostachia"†	Prairie blazing star	"Indians and others" of Lower Missouri?	Root? to treat gonorrhea. Roots to treat Commanche swollen testiles; Kindscher, p. 138, citing Carlson and Jones	James 1966: 129
Lycopodium complanatum*	Groundcedar	Blackfoot	Decoction of plant for VDs	Johnston 1987:16

Table 2, continued

Scientific Name	Common Name	Tribe	Medical Summary	Source
Menispermum canadense	Common moonseed		Syphilis, Krochmal; VD, Strandley‡	
Phytolacca americana	American pokeweed		[Not collected or documented in Dakotas] Syphilis Steinmetz‡	
Plantago major	Common plantain		Gonorrhea, Burkhill 1966;‡	
Polygonum aviculare	Prostrate knotweed		Introduced plant. Chanchroid, Keys; Gonorrhea, Nas; VD, Bliss‡	
*Pseudotsuga menziesii**	Douglas fir	Montana Indians	Spring bud decoction for certain VDs. [Not documented or collected in Dakotas.] VD Eb24:305‡	Blankinship 1905:20
Rumex crispus	Curly dock		Introduced by Europeans. Gilmore, p. 25.	
Sambucus canadensis	Common elderberry			
Sanguinaria canadensis	Bloodroot			
Smilax (cites *aristolochiifolia*, but others are found in the flora)	Sarsaparilla		Introduced plant	
Stillingia sylvatica	Queen's-delight		Southern & South-Central states. Not documented or collected in Dakotas. Syphilis, Krochmal, Standley, Steinmetz‡	
Symphoria racemosa†	"Blue wood" [Not in USDA plant list]	"Natives" of Lower Missouri	Decoction of root to treat syphilis	James 1966: 129
Tephrosia virginiana	Virginia tephrosia, goat's rue		Not documented or collected in Dakotas. Syphilis Krochmal‡ Folk remedy for syphilis, Kindscher, p. 285, citing Duke 1985.	
Trifolium pratense	Red clover		Introduced plant	
Urtica dioica	Stinging nettle		"Native and introduced"?	

* From http://herb.umd.umich.edu/herb/searc.pl, accessed June 22, 2006
† From James (1966:129)
‡ Notes from James Duke's Phytochemical and Ethnobotanical Databases. http://www.ars-grin.gov/duke/ Accessed June 23, 2006.

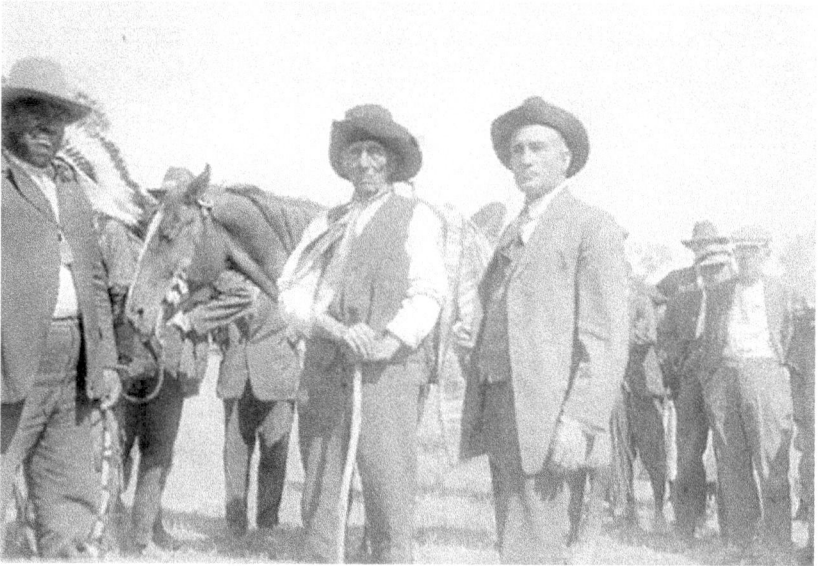

Figure 19. Melvin R. Gilmore (right foreground), University of Michigan ethnobotoanist, among the Arikara in 1918. Despite such fieldwork among the Arikara, his classic publication, *Uses of Plants by the Indians of the Upper Missouri River Region*, excludes mention of either the Arikara or traditional treatments for venereal diseases among other tribes. (Used with permission of Bentley Historical Library, University of Michigan's permission.)

Although the Arikara may or may not have used these medicinal plants, the list does provide an important perspective on plant use for medicinal purposes. It indicates a widespread interest and use of healing plants. Considering the aboriginal trade network and its exchange of information and materials across the Plains, it is likely that the Arikara were aware of many of these same plants and their properties, at least those that neighboring tribes employed.

A more direct approach to traditional Arikara medicinal plant use might come from ethnobotanical inventories documenting their use of plants and pharmacological assessments of those plants. Many ethnobotanical inventories were conducted by well-trained investigators using knowledgeable informants during the late 19th and early 20th centuries. Most notably on the Plains, Melvin R. Gilmore (1991) published information from Omaha, Ponca, Pawnee and Teton

Dakota informants (Fig. 19). Unfortunately no extensive inventory of medicinal plant uses has been published for the Arikara. And even Gilmore's detailed list of plant used by other Plains tribes omits specific mention of venereal disease or its treatments. That absence, in itself, is remarkable. Every society has treatments for what ails its members, whatever the efficacy of the treatments. The Arikara, Omaha, Ponca, Pawnee and Teton Dakota must have had treatments for venereal diseases. Perhaps this omission is due to Gilmore's, his informants' or his editors' prudishness. Whatever the cause—or causes—this omission is unfortunate and leads researchers to wonder what other sensitive information went unreported in the Plains Indian ethnobotanical literature.

The third approach to understanding traditional Arikara medicinal plants involves historic accounts, some of which we have presented in previous chapters. The traders and travelers who stopped at the Leavenworth villages made many observations, including those related to the Arikara's health and traditional medicines. There are several visitors who observed such uses.

Trudeau (1914:460-461), the St. Louis school master who lived with the Arikara as a trader during the summer of 1795, wrote "The Indians cure themselves of it [venereal disease] very easily. They showed me some who six months ago were rotting away who are now perfectly cured." Another version (Smith 1936:567) goes "This [venereal disease] is very frequent among them; but the Indians cure it by decoctions of certain roots. I have seen some that were rotten with it, cured in six months." Trudeau noted both the presence and frequency of venereal disease, as well its effective treatment using roots of unspecified plant or plants in decoctions. Trudeau did not identify the plants, an absence that may have been from his lack of formal botanical training—school master or not.

Botanist John Bradbury, on the other hand, did have botanical training, interest and employment. When he visited the Arikara villages in 1811, he had been hired to collect American plants by the Liverpool Botanical Society. As part of his extended US field trip, he noted the local flora as well as some aspects of Arikara ethnobotany. On June 14th, while walking through the upper Leavenworth village accompanying barrister Brackenridge, he (Bradbury 1904:132) was "accosted" by an Arikara healer who was treating an ill boy—most likely the same child Brackenridge described (see quotation above). The Arikara doctor believed that Bradbury was a healer because the medicine man had seen Bradbury collecting plants. He was not the first Native American to mistake a botanist for a traditional healer.

Indigenous traditional medicine so often employed plants that collecting plants was associated with doctors and healing. In some cases, the right to collect certain plants and the rituals involved with gathering medicinal plants were limited to specific Arikara medicine societies and even certain members of those societies who held specific powers (Curtis 1907-1930, 5:64)

The Arikara medicine man showed Bradbury the plants that he used, and Bradbury, ever the dutiful botanist and chronicler, identified those plants in the medicine man's bag, noting details of those plants (Bradbury 1904:133; see Table 3).

Bradbury idetified a plant the Arikara used to treat scalds (cattail). He also noted plants in the Arikara medicine man's bundle that more recent botanists identified as used to treat rheumatism and other ailments (sage), cramps and headaches (wallflower), fever and other illnesses (milkvetch). Most importantly for our purposes, Bradbury observed in the bundle what he identified as "*rudibeckia purpurea.*" More about that important plant in a moment.

It is possible that Bradbury, the botanist, over-emphasized the plants in the Arikara physician's bundle to the detriment of other

Table 3. Bradbury's list of plants in Arikara medicine man's bundle, June 14, 1811.

Bradbury's Identification	Notations*	Bradbury's Comments	Gilmore's Medicinal Summary†	Kindscher's Summary‡
Typha palustris Reedmace	Typha cattail; *T. palustris* is common species name, but none currently associated with cattail genus. Reedmace refers to cattails and bulrushes	Arikara used for burns and scalds	Typha "used for burns and scalds" p.12.	Cattail
Artemisia sp.	Various sagebrushes, sageworts, and wormwoods	Plant common on prairie, Hunters call it "hyssop"	Relieve fevers, rheumatism, irregular menstruation, stomach problems, exorcising evil spirits, p. 82-3.	--
Wall-flower. Cf. *Cheiranthus erysimoides*	Genus includes wallflowers; no species by this name	Greatest quantity of all of shaman's plants	--	Identifies as *Erysimum asperum,* western wallflower, used for cramps and headache, p. 244-5.
Astragalus	Genus of milkvetch	Two new species	*A. caroliniana* febrifuge for children, p. 39.	*A. caroliniana* Used for chest & backpains, appetite loss, spitting blood, cuts, p. 65-7.
Rudbeckia purpurea	Now *Echinacea purpurea,* eastern purple coneflower. But species not in South Dakota. [More likey *E. angustifolia,* the only *E.* native to the state]	Roots in shaman's bag; Canadians use to treat VD	*E. angustifolia* antidote for snake and other bites, headache, toothache, enlarged glands, burns, p. 79.	*E. angustifolia* widely used plant. Toothache, stomachache, sore eye, cough, colds, p. 86-8.

* From USDA Natural Resources Conservation Service's plant name search, accessed June 8, 2006.
† From Melvin R. Gilmore's *Uses of Plants by the Indians of the Missouri River Region*, 1991.
‡ From Kelly Kindscher's *Medicinal Wild Plants of the Prairie: An Ethnobotanical Guide*, 1992.

materials and rituals that may also have been used. Plants, after all, were Bradbury's passion—as well as his employment. There may have been minerals and perhaps animal parts in the medicine man's materia medica in addition to the plants—not to mention the use of chants, incantations and physical manipulations previously described by Brackenridge.

Bradbury's companion for the walk, Brackenridge (1906:117), however, supported Bradbury's emphasis on plants, saying the "simples" the medicine man showed them were "common plants with some medical properties." Unfortunately, neither he nor Bradbury indicated any specific treatment for venereal disease at that time—or any disease for that matter, except wounds.

As far as we have been able to determine, no early traveler, trader, or 20th century ethnobotanist noted the plants that the Arikara used to treat venereal diseases. There is some intriguing evidence, however, that suggests what local plants may have been employed for such purposes and indications of their means of preparation. That account follows.

In mid-July 1811, about a month after his consultation with the Arikara medicine man, botanist Bradbury (1904:180), who apparently had traveled into Mandan territory by then, wrote the following:

> I was not surprised on learning that at least two-thirds of our Canadians had experienced unpleasant consequences from their intercourse with the squaws, not withstanding which the traffic before mentioned continued.... I found some of the Canadians digging up roots, with which I understood they made a decoction, and used it as a drink. They mostly preferred the roots of *rudbeckia purpurea*, and sometimes those of *houstonia longiflolia*.

Concerning the plants Bradbury identified as being used to treat, in his words, the "unpleasant consequences," *Houstonia longifolia* (longleaf summer bluet) is a species that is still recognized today. The plant grows through the southeastern, northeastern and Midwestern states, including eastern portions of North Dakota, but apparently has not been collected as far west as the Missouri River, where the Mandan and Arikara villages were located (http://plants.usda.gov/java/nameSearch, accessed June 8, 2006).

The other plant that Bradbury saw his Canadians using to treat venereal disease he identified as "*rudbeckia purpurea*." Recall that while consulting with the Arikara medicine man, Bradbury noted roots of this same plant in the physician's medicine bundle.

That taxon was established by Linnaeus in 1753 (Foster 1985:2) and is now designated *Echinacea purpurea* (eastern purple coneflower). As the common name implies, the plant is limited in geographic distribution to the eastern and Midwestern US; the closest records of the taxon being collected to the Northern Plains are from Colorado, Iowa and Wisconsin (http://plants.usda.gov/java/nameSearch, accessed June 8, 2006). The plant Bradbury saw, based on geographic location, was more likely *E. angustifolia* (narrow leaf purple coneflower; Fig. 20), a common member of the Composite Family, growing in a broad north-to-south swath across the middle states. This taxon was established in 1836 (Foster 1985:2), 25 years after Bradbury's Arikara visit. Despite this use among his Canadians, Bradbury did not consider the plant especially noteworthy, omitting it from his "Catalogue of Some of the More Rare or Valuable Plants" that he collected on his journey (Bradbury 1904:317-320).

Other observers, however, thought the plant singular; several of them noted uses of *Echinacea* for treatment of venereal diseases, perhaps including Lewis and Clark. Cutright (1969:122, 408) suggests that the captains sent a few pounds of the root to Thomas Jefferson from Ft. Mandan in April 1805. Called "white wood of the

105

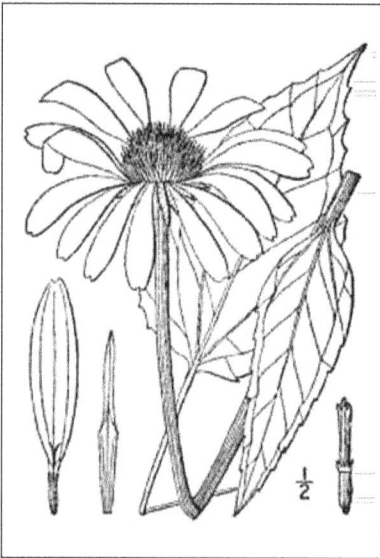

Figure 20. Purple coneflower (*Echinacea angustifolia*). Roots of the plant were likely used to treat the symptoms of venereal disease by numerous individuals, including some members of Bradbury's group. (Used with permission of USDA-NRCS PLANTS Database; and Britton, N.L., and A. Brown. 1913. *Illustrated Flora of the Northern States and Canada*. Vol. 3: 475.)

prairie" and believed to be purple coneflower, the plant merited a separate letter to Jefferson noting it as a cure for the bites of "Mad Dogs[,] Snkes &c" (Clark in Chuinard 1979:271). The sample was recommended for testing under the careful eye of the Philadelphia Philosophical Society, although it is unclear if such testing occurred, and if it did what the results were.

Other journalists also thought the plant noteworthy, particularly in the treatment of venereal diseases (from Foster 1985). The Delaware used *E. purpurea* for advanced venereal disease (Foster 1985:13). John King (1852) used *"Rudbeckia" purpurea* for syphilis (in Foster 1985:14). The label for Meyer's Blood Purifier (1880s), which included *E. angustifolia*, claimed it to be "a powerful drug as an Alternative and Antiseptic in all tumorous and Syphilitic indications;..." (in Foster 1985:15). Goss of Chicago praised the plant as remedy for both gonorrhea and syphilis (in Foster 1985: 17). So purple coneflower roots, most likely those of the narrow-leaved purple coneflower, were probably those prepared and used by Bradbury's Canadians as a treatment for venereal disease as well as many other groups later in the 19th century.

From Bradbury's and Trudeau's chronicles, we are led to believe that venereal disease among the Arikara was mild and easily cured using prepared roots. In contrast, there was the irascible Tabeau's perspective.

Tabeau wrote, "These Savages are too ignorant and too lazy to profit from the gifts of nature and to find in plants remedies for their ailments. They do not know one purgative root as this treatment is not in use" (Abel 1939:183). He continued discussing blood-letting, supernatural causes of illnesses, medicine men and their curing ceremonies as well as sorcery, without further mention of wild plant remedies.

In summary, there were apparently many, varied and inventive treatments for venereal disease by the Northern Plains' traditional healers. There is, however, no published Arikara ethnobotanical information from the late 19th or early 20th century related to venereal disease—or any other prominent Plains Indian group, for that matter. But several historic accounts suggest that venereal disease was effectively treated with a decoction of locally available roots, most likely *Houstonia longifolia* and *Echinacea angustifolia*, the latter having been used more frequently and by non-Arikara groups. The results of the Leavenworth Site skeletal and dental studies are consistent with the writings of Trudeau and Bradbury, inconsistent with those of the contrarian Tabeau. If syphilis were present, it seems to have been treatable with effective remedies that the Arikara knew.

Different Mortuary Treatment for Afflicted

Another explanation for the discrepancy between historic documents and Arikara skeletons concerns a limitation of the archaeological record. As inventive and clever as archaeologists are, they typically recover materials that are easily located or accidentally found. The obscure and hidden, the sparse and unusual typically remain lost and unknown to archaeology. This assertion may explain our mystery.

In their classic study of the Leavenworth Site skeletons, Bass et al. (1971:160-161) noted that too few skeletons were recovered archaeologically from the Leavenworth Site cemeteries to represent all of the deaths that must have occurred while the site was occupied. To reach this conclusion, they estimated the number of Arikara deaths at the Leavenworth Site. They considered the number of skeletons found, the years the villages were occupied, and an annual death rate. With that information, they contrasted the estimated number of Arikara deaths during the villages' occupancy with the number of skeletons that were archaeologically recovered. And they found a marked discrepancy.

Bass et al. (1971) estimated that the number of skeletons from the Leavenworth Site numbered 350 to 400. To derive this estimation, they considered the number of skeletons excavated from the Leavenworth cemeteries by professional and amateur archaeologists as well as a few hard-to-find skeletons that may have been missed by the excavators.

The years the villages were occupied were the next critical element. Based largely on Wedel's (1955) interpretation of historic accounts and archaeological evidence, they (Bass et al. 1971:160-161) concluded that the Arikara occupied the Leavenworth Site for 28 years, from 1803 to 1832 with two or three years' vacancy during those decades.

Finally they calculated the average annual death rate based on the estimated number of skeletons at the site (350 to 400 skeletons) and the number of years (28 years) the site was occupied

(Bass et al. 1971:160-161). The number of deaths per year averaged remarkably low: 12.5 to 14.3, depending on the number of burials estimated previously.

When the estimated village population based on death rates and recovered skeletons were compared with the historic accounts of the village populations, there was a marked contrast. The number of Leavenworth villagers was approximately 2,000 individuals based on Lewis and Clark's estimation of the number of warriors and other villagers. By 1830 the population estimation was somewhat higher: 2-4,000 (Holder 1970:30). These estimations of the Leavenworth population were nearly ten times the number of individuals expected based on the number of cemetery burials, the period the village was occupied, and death rates presented above. Bass et al. (1971) concluded that many of the Leavenworth Site dead must have been buried elsewhere or corpses disposed of otherwise than in the nearby archaeologically excavated cemeteries. They delved little into possible reasons for these omissions from cemetery burial other than establishing the facts.

To make these calculations, Bass et al. (1971) were forced to assume several things. They assumed that all deaths in the villages—or at least a large proportion of them— were buried in the cemeteries and those interments continued throughout the occupation period.

A death rate of 5 percent per year would require only a population of only 208 to 238 persons to produce the calculated average 12.5 or 14.3 deaths per year, not the 2000 or more residents that were said to live there. Similar calculations can be made for a higher death rate. A death rate of even 6 percent per year, for instance, would require a population of only 250 to 281 to produce 12.5 or 14.3 deaths per year. Even this population size is much too small compared with the historic Arikara's numbers. How is this discrepancy explained?

One possibility is related to our proposed explanation. Perhaps the Arikara with the marked lesions associated with tertiary syphilis as well as other afflicted Arikara were excluded from burial in the normal Leavenworth cemeteries. Perhaps they were buried elsewhere, thus these syphilitic individuals were among the skeletons that Bass et al. (1971) indicate were not recovered by the 20th century archaeologists.

The Arikara story of a scalped man's plight is relevant to this conjecture. (See Parks' 1982 careful analysis for more details of this tale.) The Arikara had several traditional tales involving a man who fell in a fight with enemies, was scalped, yet survived the ordeal. Because of his mutilation, the scalped man was viewed as "ruined"— no longer human—and shunned by Arikara society. Forced to live a solitary life among spirits, he was often depicted as inhabiting a hillside cave. He lived furtively, traveling at night, subsisting by theft of village goods as well as other antisocial means. On the other hand, the scalped man was often imbued with supernatural powers, powers that included providing supplicants with materials, including provisions, horses, eagles or scalps—though presumably not his own already-missing scalp. He also provided power or esoterica related to "medicine." He was depicted variously as a legend, mythical figure, or bogeyman, whose existence was used to make children behave. Despite these powers, the scalped man, according to the tales, died alone, his body either not found or if found, buried in an isolated spot, and thus excluded from cemetery burial.

Before continuing with this explanation, a related subject is in order. In this work, we have been using archaeological skeletons from the 19th century Arikara Leavenworth Site to assess historical documents. Not only can skeletal remains be used to amplify historical accounts, skeletons can also be used to assess and elaborate traditional tales, in this case that of the scalped man.

Skulls emerging from the earth may have circular abnormalities. Two explanations are possible: scalping and syphilis. To make sense of the differences, we need to consider, for a moment, anatomical structures.

The bony skull has three layers: an inner and an outer layer, both of hard, dense bone, and a middle layer of spongy bone, filled with small veins. Over the dome of the skull are two layers of tough, fibrous membrane. The inner layer (the periosteum) is tightly adherent to the bone. The outer layer (the galea aponeurotica) is separated from the inner membrane by a cleft, which enables the scalp to be moved back and forth about a centimeter.

Oxygen and nourishment is brought to the scalp by superficial branches of the exterior carotid artery. The "used" blood drains through hundreds of small veins into the spongy middle layer of the skull bone.

The usual technique of scalping involves severing the galea aponeurotica and periosteum, down to the bone, and ripping the soft tissue away from the skull. If the victim is already dead, there is, of course, no healing process. In the few victims who survive this ordeal, there are five stages of recovery. First, the outer hard layer of the skull and the spongy layer, deprived of nourishment and exposed to the air, both die. Second, granulation tissue begins to form, separating live bone from dead. Third, the dead bone is shed, leaving only the inner hard layer of the skull to protect the brain. Fourth, new bone begins to grow, filling in the hole. Finally, the defect is covered with new skin and with new bone, which never quite fill the defect, leaving a depression, a shallow dent of the size and shape of the original scalping (Hamperl 1967).

The skull lesions of syphilis, termed caries sicca (literally "dry cavities") look much different. They usually begin as clusters of pits in the bone. These clusters begin to fuse, creating larger pits, with ragged sharp edges, as though rat gnawn. The outer layers of the bone are destroyed and, in a later stage, replaced along the margins of the defect by an outer layer of defective bone. The lesions may be as small as an inch across or large enough to involve the whole skull vault.

These different appearances help the archaeologist and osteologist seeking to distinguish between a scalped skull and a syphilitic one.

There are several archaeologically recovered scalped skulls and their contexts shed light on Arikara society and its relation to scalped individuals (see Hollimon and Owsley 1994:350-351 for a summary). Some of these scalped survivors have been attributed to historic Arikara, others to prehistoric or protoArikara societies. They include an adolescent female, dating approximately AD 1650-1725 from the Sully Site in central South Dakota. Her lesions were actively healing at the time of death (Hollimon and Owsley 1994:350-351). Another healing scalping occurs in an adult (50-60 years) female from the Spiry-Eklo Site, near the Leavenworth Site but below the Grand River, dating approximately 1700AD (Hamperl and Laughlin 1959).

The site with greatest number of healed scalpings is the 14th century Crow Creek Site, in south-central South Dakota, where at least 486 individuals were killed in a massacre and their bodies buried in the dry moat surrounding the village (Willey 1990; Willey and Emerson 1993). Among the hundreds of massacre victim skulls were two that apparently had survived previous scalping ordeals only to be killed later during wholesale village slaughter. One was an adult (25-45 years) female (Box-Bag 107-1; Skull 264), and the other was an adult with no sex identification or more specific age identification (Box-Bag 41-2, Skull 13). Because those two skulls were found among the massacre victims' remains, it appears that the previously scalped persons were included in mainstream Arikara society, died in the massacre and were interred in the mass grave.

All of these archaeological examples contrast with the oral Arikara tale involving the banishment and shunning of the "non-human" scalped man. Concerning the presence of Arikara scalping survivors in normal mortuary contexts—at least not buried in an isolated place—and the Arikara tale of the scalped man, Hollimon and Owsley (1994:352) write "Perhaps the banishment [of the scalped man] was more typical of the early historic period or an age or gender association is indicated (that is, scalped women were not exiled)." Bones suggest complexity—by time period, age and sex—to the Arikara's dealings with scalped people. The tale of the scalped man does not.

Surviving scalping must have been extraordinarily rare. When you are down in battle, you are normally down as well as out. And exclusion of the few scalped men from burial in an Arikara cemetery would have had little impact on cemetery burial counts and their demography. But their exclusion from cemetery burial has relevance to our argument concerning the Arikara, syphilis and the Leavenworth skeletons.

Here is how the plight of the scalped man may relate to our mystery. When a person was scalped and survived the trauma, the blood vessels to scalp tissue were often severed. As all biological tissues, scalp requires the blood to carry nutrients and oxygen to the cells and remove wastes and carbon dioxide. Lacking the arteries and veins that transport blood, the adjacent tissues die. They become "necrotic."

The Arikara may have considered the cranial vault necrosis associated with surviving scalping similar to the appearance of caries sicca associated with the classic syphilitic cranial vault. Further, some of those individuals—whether scalped or syphilitic—may have been shunned and forced to live a solitary life separate from the rest of Arikara society. When they died, they may have been excluded from burial in the Arikara cemeteries and thus not archaeologically recovered. If our explanation follows, then shunned syphilis victims were excluded from cemetery burial and not readily available for archaeological recovery, thus no syphilitic skeletons were included in the collections.

Summary

There are a number of possible historic and ethnographic explanations for the discrepancy between the historic accounts and the skeletal remains. We presented three of them.

It is possible, although unlikely, that there was a mistaken diagnosis of the ailments by the 19th century chroniclers. This explanation seems unlikely considering the explorers' background and knowledge. It also seems unlikely considering other independent reports from the period that echo Lewis and Clark's identifications. Venereal disease was almost certainly present among the historic Arikara.

A second possibility is that the Arikara had effective traditional remedies for venereal diseases. It is possible that the Arikara medicine men, their curing ceremonies, or medicines were effective in treating venereal diseases. Along these lines, it is possible that their use of medicinal plants, such as purple coneflower roots, healed or at least mitigated the effects of venereal diseases.

A final explanation is that there was different mortuary treatment of those afflicted with venereal disease than the unaffected, thus making the afflicted unrecoverable by the archaeologists.

These explanations involve historic and ethnographic causes. There is, in addition, another suite of possible explanations. Those include biological and skeletal explanations and are considered in the next chapter.

7. Skeletal and Biological
Explanations

In the previous chapter we considered historic and ethnographic explanations for the mystery of the bones. It is time to turn to more tangible explanations, those spotlighting the skeletal system and other biological parameters.

There are five biologically oriented explanations. First, the osteological conclusions could be erroneous: the 19th century Arikara and their skeletons had venereal disease, but for one reason or another the illness was not identified. It is also possible that the Arikara were biologically adapted to syphilis, thus the skeletons did not manifest the disease. Another explanation involves the relatively young age of the 19th century Arikara; syphilitic skeletal lesions require time to develop and if the Arikara were too short-lived, they may not have lived long enough to show the effects of the disease. In addition to the time requirements, there are limitations of the skeleton to manifest syphilis. And finally it is also possible that the disease, syphilis, or its manifestations may have changed since the early 1800s. Each of these explanations is considered.

Erroneous Osteological Conclusions

Just as the ethnographic and historic documents may be inaccurate or we have misinterpreted them, a similar case can be made for the interpretations of the Arikara bones. To paraphrase the adage, "bones don't lie, but liars do bones." It is possible that the osteologists missed the diagnosis for one of several reasons.

Syphilis is the protean disease, with many and varied manifestations, especially in its tertiary stage. This enormous variation in disease manifestations is not only true of soft tissues, but also true of skeletal involvement, variation that potentially confounds identification of the disease. Even if we limit ourselves to considering classic skeletal manifestations of syphilis, there are additional problems.

Acquired venereal syphilis' skeletal hallmarks are caries sicca and saber shins. Either indicator may be obscured, however, by the vicissitudes of preservation. And some of the Leavenworth Site cemeteries (especially the eastern-most cemetery) had poor bone preservation. Some bones preserved so poorly there that they were the consistency of oatmeal. If caries sicca or saber shins were present in those bones, they may have been obscured by deterioration in the ground.

As if complications from poor bone preservation were not limiting enough, there is the additional issue of dental wear on the teeth's occlusal surfaces. The most distinctive indicators of congenital syphilis are Hutchinson's incisors and mulberry molars. Such occlusal surface malformations, however, may be obscured by dental attrition (Goff 1967:286). Many traditional groups have a diet with coarse, abrasive materials in prepared foods, resulting in extensive occlusal attrition. Attrition first grinds off the highest, most exposed enamel on the teeth's occlusal surfaces, including cusps. The occlusal surfaces and cusps are the parts that are most likely to show notching and the convoluted cusps associated with congenital syphilis. As

116

attrition continues, the next layer of the tooth—dentin—is exposed and abraded. Because dentin is less durable than enamel, it wears faster than enamel. As attrition continues, the surface wears toward the centrally located tooth pulp, where nerves, blood and lymph vessels reside. When attrition breaches the pulp cavity, microbes have access to the tooth's interior. Once there, infection and abscessing occur and the tooth is lost. Crown attrition and antemortem tooth loss have implications for identifying congenital syphilis among the Leavenworth Site skeletons.

The Leavenworth Site teeth had significant wear, as indicated by attrition exposing tooth pulp and subsequent tooth abscessing (Ubelaker 1971:193), at least in some middle-aged adult Leavenworth skeletons. This attrition and abscessing may have obscured or eliminated some teeth with diagnostic characteristics of syphilis. It is especially appropriate to our discussion because the enamel resulting from congenital syphilis is of poor quality (Fournier 1884, cited in Powell and Cook 2005:28) and less resistant to attrition, thus more prone to caries, abscess and loss. Despite these limitations, at least some of the younger Leavenworth individuals' teeth should have shown indications of congenital syphilis: distinctive mulberry molars or Hutchinson's incisors, indicating congenital syphilis. But they did not. So, this explanation alone does not explain the absence of syphilis-modified teeth.

Even if the bones and teeth were present and well preserved, it is possible that osteologists observed but misinterpreted the lesions. This error is analogous to historic accounts noting but misinterpreting disease.

Shermis's description of the Leavenworth skeleton's paleopathology is amenable to assessing this possibility. Shermis (1969) provided both descriptions and identifications of the diseases he observed. His descriptions are useful to appraise the possibility that syphilis was present in the Arikara skeletons, but he identified them as resulting from other diseases. There are two of these "questionable calls."

Leavenworth Site Skeleton 68 (middle-aged male) had, in addition to several healed fractures, a hole through the right scapular spine (Shermis 1969:15-16). Shermis recognized that the hole may or may not have resulted from injury and may have been caused by a focal infection (Shermis 1969:15). He also noted alterations to both clavicles, which he attributed to trauma alone (Shermis 1969:16). Instead of these alterations indicating injuries, it is possible that both the scapula and clavicles lesions resulted from a bone-altering infection and that infection may have been treponemal in origin.

Leavenworth Site Skeleton 258 (young adult male) had bone destruction and remodeling of the distal metatarsals (Shermis 1969: 35-36). Although the analyst identified the defects as the results of rheumatoid arthritis, it is possible that alterations were caused by a treponemal infection and the osteological expressions were one of many unusual manifestations of the disease.

Shermis identified other skeletons with lesions that might possibly be associated with venereal disease, including an ankle of an adolescent (Skeleton 202) that showed the effects of infection (Shermis 1969:45-46). But the two cases presented above are the most probable ones. If any of these three—or any others, for that matter—originated from venereal disease, then there is skeletal evidence supporting the early travelers' and traders' reports. That, however, is not how the original analyst identified the diseases, despite his familiarity with the historic accounts and their reports of venereal disease.

If syphilis was present but no skeletal lesions were present, how do we explain the absence of bone manifestations? Is it possible that the Arikara had some genetic resistance to the disease?

Constitutional Resistance to Disease

Some infectious diseases occurred among Native Americans in PreColumbian times, and this continent's natives, as all people, adapted biologically during their millennia of exposure to the pathogens. Such is the nature of evolutionary change. Non-natives, who had not been previously exposed and had no such adaptations to the indigenous microbes, were more vulnerable to the ravages of the diseases.

Varying susceptibility of different groups to the same disease has often been noted. In these cases, the biological virulence of the pathogen seems to be similar in all groups, but susceptibility differs from one group to another. So, individuals from one group may express relatively light and inconsequential symptoms when exposed to a particular disease, and individuals in another group may express devastating effects of the same disease. It is that differing susceptibility among populations that is of interest here.

Population Decline in Native Americans

When Europeans reached the Americas, Native Americans had greater susceptibility to some of the common European diseases. The most notorious of those introduced Old World diseases were the so-called "crowd" and "childhood" infections that caused severe epidemics. These diseases included smallpox, measles, chicken pox, diphtheria, typhoid fever, cholera, and malaria.

Combined with other impacts resulting from contact with Europeans, these diseases had devastating effects on many Native American groups. The most easily quantifiable and most frequently employed means of documenting these processes is population decline. Most often population decline is presented from the time of first European contact until the lowest population number (nadir). For North America as a whole, Native American population is estimated to have decreased from first contact to nadir by 78 percent, with the Great Plains suffering a slightly less decrease of 69 percent (Ubelaker 2006:699, table 4). Most of the regional nadirs occurred about 1900, and since then the Native American populations have been increasing.

Take the Arikara as an example of a continent-wide nose-dive in population numbers. The earliest Arikara population estimation was by Trudeau. For the pre-contact, pre-epidemic Arikara, he estimated there were 4,000 warriors or about 16,000 Arikara altogether (Figure 21). By 1795, following the early epidemics and when Trudeau was living with the Arikara, they were reduced to only an eighth of that number, approximately 500 warriors. This number is comparable to Tabeau's and Lewis and Clark's estimations in 1804 of 2,000 to 3,000 Arikara. And the population continued to decline for another century until 1905 as disease and disruption ripped the fabric of Arikara life (Parks 2001:387-388, table 3). From the estimated pre-contact Arikara population (16,000) to nadir of 379 in 1905, there was a decrease of 97 percent. This figure is a phenomenal one. Perhaps Trudeau's estimation of the pre-contact Arikara population was an overstatement. When the more conservative Lewis and Clark figure (2,000) is employed, there was a decrease of 81 percent—about the percentage estimated for the overall continent-wide decrease. Whichever figure is employed, the results are similar: a tragic drop in Arikara population occurred.

Most of this population decline is attributed to deaths from epidemics. Smallpox hit the Arikara three times in the 1770s as well as in the 1830s, 1850s and twice in the 1860s. The smallpox epidemic of 1837, it was claimed, killed about half of the Arikara (Chardon in Abel 1932:138). Note, however, our Figure 21 does not show such a drastic decrease, not in that period. In addition to smallpox, other infectious diseases, such as measles and cholera, struck the Arikara in

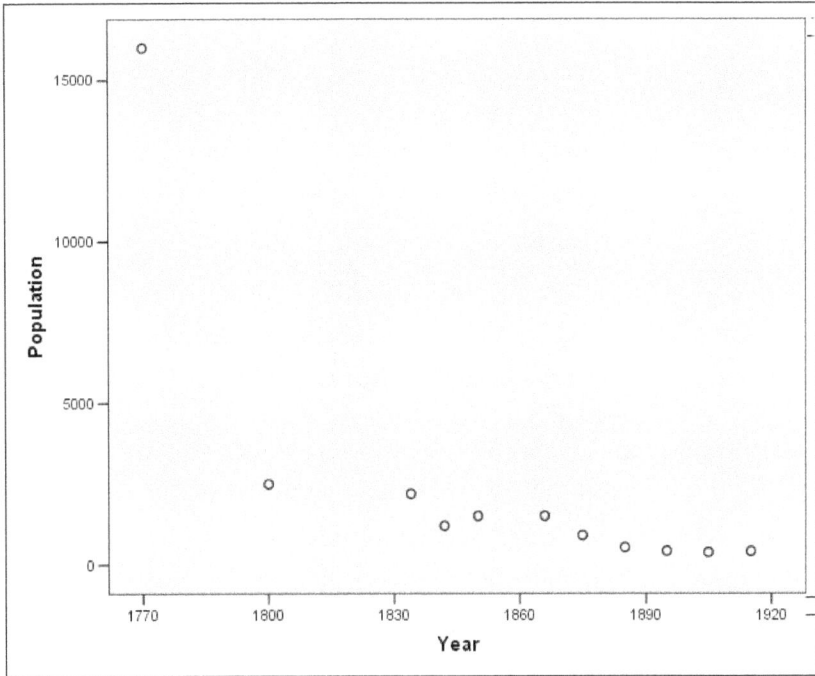

Figure 21. Arikara population decline from the mid-18th century through the early 20th century. (Data from Parks 2001: 387-388, table 3).

the mid-1800s. And in addition to the epidemic diseases, warfare and interpersonal violence, social disintegration and culture change pummeled the Arikara, causing a drastic population decrease (Owsley 1992:83).

Smallpox

Smallpox is an excellent example of this terrible situation. Europeans and Asians had been exposed to the disease for millennia and had developed some biological resistance, although not immunity, to it. Europeans had a genetically built-in biological resistance buffering them from this disease as well as cultural means of dealing with the disease.

Smallpox is caused by a virus spread by droplets from an infected person, usually transmitted by entering the next victim's nose or mouth. Variola major has severe symptoms, often resulting in fatalities as high as 20% of its victims even in recent times (Fenner et al. 1988:3). Following exposure, the incubation period is usually 10 to 14 days (Fenner et al. 1988:5). The most notable symptom is raised skin pustules, appearing 12 to 18 days after exposure. Before the appearance of the rash, which later develops into pustules, a number of other early symptoms occur. The most frequent early symptoms are high fever, muscle pain, malaise and headache, although convulsions, delirium and vomiting may occur (Fenner et al. 1988:5-6). But it is the pustules that are the diagnostic symptom, hence the disease's name.

By the seventh day following the earliest symptoms, the skin lesions form pustules. The lesions are distributed in a distinctive pattern; they are greatest in the face and limbs—especially on the more distal portions of the limbs, and least on the trunk (Fenner et al. 1988:21). The lesions gradually scab over and heal, although scars often persist long afterwards as pockmarks (Fenner et al. 1988: 49).

Contrasted with variola major, variola minor has milder symptoms and lower fatality rates, about 1 percent deaths in recent times (Fenner et al. 1988:3). The symptoms are similar to those associated with variola major, but generally milder than the more virulent form of the disease. Rashes are less severe, temperatures are lower, and there is a faster course of the disease (Fenner et al. 1988:38-39). Complications of either form of the disease, however, might include skin infections via the pustules, blindness, arthritis and limb deformities (Fenner et al. 1988:48, 50)

As late as 1967 it was estimated that smallpox killed 2 million people worldwide each year (Pratt 1999:177). But thanks to what has been described both as "completely successful and extraordinarily cost-effective" and the "world's most successful programme" (Pratt 1999:177), the virus is no longer considered a threat. Smallpox was officially declared eradicated by 1977. It was not considered a threat, that is, until 2001 when the possibility that terrorists might use the virus for their purposes emerged. The more things change, the more they stay the same! But back to the past.

In the 18th and 19th centuries, smallpox spread through previously unexposed Plains Native American communities with catastrophic effects. Whole villages, whole tribes fell ill simultaneously. "Virgin soil epidemics," they are termed because the population is inexperienced with the disease.

Amerindians had little biological resistance to smallpox as well as many other EuroAsian diseases, so the epidemic diseases spread quickly, laying low whole groups at the same time. All ages and both sexes were susceptible, leading to disintegration of day-to-day village life, rupturing social networks and responsibilities. With few healthy villagers present, simple but essential daily chores, such as fetching water and preparing meals, went undone and malaise descended. Native Americans were not unique in such biological and social responses. A similar set of catastrophic events occurred when the Black Death swept Medieval Europe.

Origin of Syphilis

In many ways, the two hemispheres were separate worlds and parallel before they collided, each with its own pathogens and health challenges. There is another direction to flow of diseases other than the Old World-to-America direction that diseases such as smallpox traveled. Although not as well known, there was an America-to-Europe spread of disease as well. And some aspects of that New World-to-Old World flow has been a matter of hot debate for five centuries.

Merbs (1992:3) claims that there were a number of diseases that were indigenous to the New World that traveled to the Old World following contact. Among the better known diseases, he lists tuberculosis, fungal infections (such as coccidioidomycosis), Rocky Mountain spotted fever, adult rheumatoid arthritis, and Lyme disease. Probably the best known—certainly the most pertinent to our discussion here—is the debate concerning the New World origin of syphilis.

If syphilis was a New World disease and natives developed resistance to the disease over many generations, as Europeans did to their indigenous diseases such as smallpox, then syphilis may have had less impact on Native Americans in the 16th and 17th centuries than it had on Europeans. Such may have been the case of syphilis among the Arikara. Botanist Bradbury (1904:180), who visited the Arikara in 1811, wrote "I had been informed by Jones and Carson of the existence of this evil [venereal disease], but found it of the mildest description, and that here, where the natives do not use spirituous liquors nor salt, it is not feared." It is possible that Arikara as well as some other Native American groups had developed a resistance to syphilis through long-term adaptation to the disease. To put Bradbury's observation in a broader context, we discuss the two competing hypothesis concerning syphilis' origin.

The Columbian Hypothesis maintains that syphilis originated in the Americas and only after 1492 and Columbus' voyages was the disease introduced to the Old World.

Columbus himself may have been one of the first victims of New World syphilis. In the memorable year 1492, he was a healthy, vigorous man of 41 years. On his second voyage he was feverish, delirious, and often blind, with intermittent memory failure. By his third voyage, all his joints were inflamed; he had auditory hallucination and believed he was a special emissary of God. On his final voyage, he had celestial visions and a voice spoke to him about the Bible. All these symptoms suggest syphilis (Lowry 2004:20).

Supporters of the Columbian Hypothesis note that the "Great pox" (contrasted with the smallpox) hit Europe in the late 1400s. It spread quickly across Asia, arriving in Japan by 1511.

Contrasted with the Columbian Hypothesis, the Pre-Columbian Hypothesis argues that syphilis originated in the Old World long before Columbus' voyages. Syphilis, this hypothesis claims, was diagnostically confused with leprosy and other diseases. Syphilis was lumped with those other diseases as a single entity, despite it being present before 1492. Finally about 1500, the diseases were recognized as separate entities, and it was the diagnostic identifications of the diseases—not a microbial infection—that spread after 1500.

With that background, we return to our argument. If syphilis originated in the New World, as the Columbian Hypothesis claims, and Native Americans had been exposed to the disease for many generations, then they may have adapted to it and have been less affected by the syphilis spirochete than the un-adapted Europeans. And if Native Americans were less affected by syphilis, then they might have had less frequent and less severe skeletal involvement.

Syphilis and ABO Blood Types

There is some intriguing biomolecular evidence involving the ABO blood system that supports this explanation. Before presenting this evidence, however, a little biological background is necessary.

The ABO blood system is the best known of all human genetic systems. It involves surface proteins of the red blood cells, those critical structures that transport oxygen to the body's tissues. These entities are antigens (immune response producers) that make antibodies. The system has three alleles (or "genes"): A, B and O. These three alleles, one from each parent, combine to form four phenotypes: A, B, AB and O. A and B are dominant over O, and codominant between themselves. These phenotypes are what people commonly refer to as their blood type.

As an aside, the positive and negatives sometimes associated with ABO blood types are inherited through different genes, called the Rh or Rhesus System. They are genetically independent and separate from the ABO system.

Because the ABO system is clinically important, its worldwide geographic distribution is relatively well known and much analyzed. This documentation involves examining the blood groups of the various indigenous people of the geographic regions—not just the many recent migrants and the current residents. Of the three blood groups in the ABO system, Allele A has an erratic distribution, being most frequent in Australia, Scandinavia, and a few Northwest Plains groups. It is least frequent among indigenous Latin Americans.

Allele B is most frequent in central Asia, being less frequent to the east and west of that area. It is nearly absent from Australia and the Americas. This relative absence from the Americas is surprising because most scholars concur that Native Americas originated from Asian ancestry. Because B is most frequent among Central Asians, Native Americans should have carried the B allele with them when they arrived in the Americas from Asia, but based on present-day Native American blood type frequencies, that situation does not seem to be the case.

On a worldwide basis, Allele O is the most common blood group. It is more frequent than either of the other ABO alleles on every continent and in nearly all populations. In Central and South America, as well as some parts of North America, it approaches 100%—to the near exclusion of A and B alleles. And that distribution is critical for our discussion.

The ABO alleles are not randomly distributed, and the reasons for that nonrandomness have intrigued anthropologists for decades. Some authorities, Alice Brues foremost among them, argued that the ABO system's immune response may make some groups more or less vulnerable to certain diseases. Such may be the case with the ABO system, and its response to cholera, plague, smallpox and—most relevant here—syphilis.

Since the 1940s, venereal syphilis has been effectively treated in all peoples with antibiotics, the first antibiotic developed being penicillin. But before the advent of antibiotics, such successes were infrequent.

In a study based on a sample from the pre-penicillin period, researchers (Vogel and Motulsky 1997; Vogel et al. 1960) found differences among syphilis-infected people based on their blood type. They discovered that people with allele O were more likely to respond favorably to treatment using neosalvarsan, an arsenic-based medicine developed in the early 20th century. Following a treatment course with neosalvarsan, individuals with blood type O were more likely to become seronegative than those individuals with A, B or AB blood types. This apparently successful treatment may indicate that the disease took a less virulent course in people with blood type O, and as a consequence of this diminished virulence, neosalvarsan was more effective with blood type O individuals than those with other blood groups.

More importantly, the same researchers found that individuals with blood types A, B and AB were 1.7 times more likely to develop tertiary syphilis (the stage when skeletal lesions appear) than those with O. So, when syphilis reduces fertility of infected mothers and increases mortality, it should be the possessors of blood types A, B and AB that are most adversely affected, and those people with O are least affected. In other words, O individuals appear to be better adapted to syphilis than individuals who are blood types A, B or AB.

How about the Arikara? How do these generalities fit them? As far as we can determine, there is no publication documenting Arikara ABO blood types. This absence, for our purposes, is an unfortunate omission.

On the other hand, there are two related tribes whose ABO blood type frequencies have been reported: Pawnee and Caddo. The Pawnee in the early 19th century lived in the Central Plains and most authorities (summarized in Parks 2001:365-366) believe the Arikara and Pawnee came from a common stock that split, based on archaeological, biological, cultural and linguistic evidence, between 1000-1500AD. The other group, the Caddo, is more distantly related to Arikara. In the early 19th century they were living in the east Texas and adjacent states. Their association with the Arikara is based mostly on linguistic inferences and the two tribes are believed to have split as much as several thousand years ago. By the late 19th century, most of the Pawnee and Caddo were "removed" and lived on reservations in Oklahoma

There, on the reservations in the mid-20th century, researchers drew blood samples from small numbers of Pawnee and Caddo. Researchers segregated "full bloods" from other admixed individuals and found that most of the full bloods were blood type A or O, very few being B or AB (Table 4, Gray and Laughlin 1960). If the 20th century Pawnee and Caddo can be assumed to be representative of the early 19th century Arikara, then the Amerindians that Lewis and Clark met possessed low frequencies of blood type B.

So, the high frequency of blood type O among 20th century Native Americans—and presumably early 19th century Arikara— may be because O confers some resistance to syphilis and/or the other treponemal diseases. As a caution, the authors of the original

Table 4. ABO blood type frequencies in 20th century Full Blood Pawnee and Caddo living in Oklahoma. (Data from Gray and Laughlin 1960).

Blood Type	Pawnee	Caddo
O	50.0	94.4
A	45.6	5.6
B	4.3	0
AB	0	0

work (Vogel and Motulsky 1997; Vogel et al. 1960) note that this interpretation assumes that at least some of the treponemal diseases were present, frequent and widespread in PreColumbian America, and that the major treponemal disease was syphilis. Those assumptions are yet to be tested.

In summary, there is the possibility that Native Americans had biological resistance to syphilis assuming they had many generations of exposure to the disease. This suggestion rests on several tangential lines of evidence. First there is the assumption of the New World origin of syphilis. Next there are the historic accounts indicating relative mild venereal symptoms among the Arikara. Then there is the possibility that blood type O is associated with some resistance to syphilis. And finally there is the observation that Native Americans have a high frequency of blood type O. These observations are intriguing lines of evidence, but the assumptions rest on an unstable foundation. Perhaps there are more substantial biological explanations for the mystery of the bones.

Arikara Too Short-Lived for Advanced Stages of Syphilis

There is another biological explanation for the discrepancy between the historic accounts concerning the presence of syphilis among the 19th century Arikara and the absence of syphilitic lesions in the Leavenworth Site skeletons. This explanation is demographic and is related to the Arikara's short life span. According to this explanation, many of the historic Arikara were susceptible to syphilis and some contracted it, but as a group they lived such short lives, dying so young, that there was not enough time for the diagnostic skeletal lesions to develop.

To examine this explanation, we first present early 19th century Arikara life expectancy using the Leavenworth Site skeletons as the foundation and include a historic account concerning elderly Arikara to flesh-out the skeletal determinations. Then we examine how much time is required once a person is infected to develop the distinctive skeletal lesions of acquired syphilis. Finally we estimate the syphilis rate in pre-penicillin populations similar to the early Arikara. These figures are required to assess this explanation and establish a basis for the section that follows this one.

Life Expectancy

Nineteenth century Arikara life expectancy, as that of many other 19th century Native Americans groups, was short. Bass et al.'s (1971:159-160) Leavenworth Site demographic data are telling along these lines. The skeletons showed a high infant and early child mortality rate. There was a 52.5% death rate for those aged 5 years and younger, indicating a life expectancy at birth of less than 5 years. Perhaps some of this Leavenworth Site youth mortality was from congenital syphilis, although, as noted above, none of the skeletons show lesions that were diagnostic of the disease. Whatever the causes, this is a remarkably high mortality with a correspondingly low life expectancy, at least when compared with contemporary populations.

The shortest present-day life expectancies are in southern Africa. Their life expectancies are in the 40s. At the opposite end of the demographic spectrum, today's longest life expectancies are 78-85 years, achieved in Japan and several wealthy microstates. Increases in life expectancy have occurred through much of history. In the US, for instance, the life expectancy in 1900 was approximately 30 years—several years less than that of current southern

Africa. Life expectancy in the US, increased to 62 years in 1985, and stood at 74.8-80.1 years in 2003. (UN Vital Statistics 2000-2004, http://unstats.un.org/unsd/demographic/products/dyb/DYB2004/Table04.pdf, accessed December 26, 2006).

So the life expectancy of the Arikara living at the Leavenworth Site was short—more accurately, it was terrible—but it was not the worst the Arikara had seen. Examining "preadult" (<15 years) mortality among the Arikara and protoArikara from other Arikara sites, Owlsey (1992:79, fig. 2) found the Leavenworth figure the next-to-the-best in his sample. Worse than Leavenworth were the 1740-1795 (Cheyenne River, Four Bear, and Leavitt sites), 1679-1733 (Larson Site) and 1600-1700 (Mobridge Site) samples. If a person could pick when and where he/she were to be born, clearly the 17th through 19th century Arikara would not be the first choice. Life was brief.

As if high infant and childhood Arikara mortality were not bad enough, it was even worse for the elderly, even the Leavenworth elderly. Because of the high childhood mortality as well as the high death rate in subsequent age stages, there were relatively few older Leavenworth adults. Bass et al. (1971:159, table 39) found only 5.6% of the skeletons lived to be 40 years or older and none of them lived to be 50 years old (Bass et al. 1971:160, table 40).

The historic accounts, however, elaborate and dispute this point concerning the elderly. According to at least one account, there were old people living in the Arikara villages. Barrister Brackenridge (1906:122), visiting the Arikara in 1811, noted

> One day, in passing through the village, I saw something brought out of a lodge in a buffaloe robe, and exposed to the sun; on approaching, I discovered it to be a human being, but so shrivelled [sic.] up, that it had nearly lost the human physiognomy: almost the only sign of life discernible, was a continual sucking its hands, and feeble moan like that of an infant. On

inquiring of the chief, he told me that he had seen it
so ever since he was a boy. He [presumably the chief]
appeared to be at least forty-five.

Brackenridge (1906:123) added that he saw other Arikara who
appeared to be almost 100 years old. So, if Brackenridge is correct,
then there were elderly adults living in the Arikara villages, something that the skeletal analyses only obliquely support at best, and
reject at worst.

Syphilis in the Bone

Returning now to the bones and what they tell, recall that the
skeletal lesions associated with acquired venereal syphilis usually
require 2 to 10 years to develop following initial exposure (Ortner
2003:279). Depending on how short-lived the Arikara were, there
may not have been enough time for syphilitic skeletal lesions to
develop. Bass et al.'s (1971:159-160, table 39) data can be employed
again, this time to estimate the number of skeletons expected to have
the disease. Summing Bass's 18-30, 31-40 and 40+ year age interval
counts, approximately one third of the Leavenworth Site sample was
adult (n=100, 35.2% of Leavenworth skeletons). This third of the
sample would have been those individuals who were or had been
sexually active and susceptible to having acquired venereal syphilis.
Over time, infected individuals would potentially express the skeletal
manifestations of the disease.

Using this number of adult skeletons from the Leavenworth Site
as a starting point, we can estimate the number of tertiary syphilitic
cases expected in the Leavenworth Site skeletal sample. Two additional figures are required before making that calculation. We must
estimate the frequency of syphilis in the Arikara population and consider the frequency of syphilis infections that affects the skeleton.

Syphilis Rates

The frequency of acquired venereal syphilis in the historic Arikara villages is, of course, unknown. No public health official examined the 19th century Arikara or drew blood to identify those carrying the disease. And of course, diagnostic tests were not available until the next century. So, estimating the Arikara syphilis rate requires other means.

To estimate the 19th century Arikara syphilis rate, we need a select set of circumstances. We turn to syphilis frequencies of groups who were screened for all syphilis cases—including the asymptomatic one. Those studies must predate public health measures, including effective treatments (such as penicillin) and prevention of the disease (such as widespread use of condoms). For these select groups, the rate of syphilis infection was between 5% (Steinbock 1976:110) and 10% (McElligott 1960 cited in Ortner 2003: 279). These figures come from European urban areas during a time predating the antibiotic period. Based on this information, then, we estimate that the adult Leavenworth Arikara villagers had a comparable syphilis rate of 5 to 10%.

Next, we return to the Leavenworth Site cemetery adult sample size. As established above, there are 100 adults in Bass's Leavenworth Site sample. With our estimated syphilis frequency of 5 to 10%, five to ten of the 100 adult skeletons should have had syphilis. This figure assumes that those with syphilis were no more likely to die than those without the disease; in other words, those individuals afflicted with syphilis were healthy enough to survive until manifestation of the disease's tertiary phase. It also requires several other assumptions that will be discussed later.

We have estimated the Arikara syphilis infection rate, the period required for skeletal lesions to develop, and the number of Leavenworth Site adult ($\geq$ 18 years) skeletons. One final estimation is required before calculating the frequency of Leavenworth Site skeletons expected to manifest syphilitic lesions. That issue is the limited nature of the skeletal system and its response to syphilis.

Limitations of Skeleton

The skeleton, while rich in some information, is notorious for its silence and ambiguity in many matters, including such important issues as age at death and disease. We first consider the problems associated with estimating age at death from the skeleton, relating it to some of the issues presented above. Then we present the problems involved with identifying disease from the skeleton. Finally we return to the issue raised in the previous section: the biological relationship between syphilis, the early 19th century Arikara, and the Leavenworth Site skeletons.

Problems with Skeletal Age Estimations

As mentioned in the previous section, Bass et al. (1971) found few older individuals in their Leavenworth Site skeletal series. Although some of the absence of the older people may be due to different mortuary treatment of the elderly (see previous chapter for that discussion), there is a biologically related alternative explanation. This explanation concerns the inaccuracy of estimating age at death from the skeleton, emphasizing limited skeletal age standards and the inaccuracy of age estimations.

Most standards used today to estimate adult skeletal age were established on three broad groups: urban US White and Black cadavers from the early 20th century, or US war dead from the mid-20th century, or medical examiner/coroner autopsies of US corpses from the late 20th century. Bass and coworkers (1971) make only general comments concerning their age estimation techniques, suggesting they used pubic symphysis morphology changes to estimate adult ages. The pubic morphology techniques most frequently employed when that analysis was conducted were Todd's standards based on a early 20th century Midwestern US cadaver series, and McKern and Stewart's phases based on US Korean War dead.

Neither of these adult age standards was based on Native American skeletons, let alone Arikara from the early 19th century. Such specialized, focused age standards are still not available today, 35 years later. But let us consider how this limitation impacts the accuracy of age estimations.

We know that the rate and timing of how people age has changed through history. Our 19th century ancestors, for instance, were old by 35 years, an age we now consider barely middle age. So, accuracy of the 20th century US standards to estimate the ages of early historic Arikara is uncertain. It is possible that early 19th century Arikara adults aged more slowly than the 20th century US groups on whom the age estimation techniques were established, and thus, those techniques tend to underestimate the historic Arikara ages. As a consequence of age underestimation, this reasoning goes, there appear to be no older Arikara skeletons, while there actually were many. Their skeletons were present. Their ages were just under-estimated by the osteologists.

An additional issue related to age estimation is how accurately older individuals' ages can be estimated even with the most appropriate age standards. There is much variation in how people age. Consider, for instance, youngsters' growth and development.

Think of a classroom full of sixth graders. Some of them are the size of children while some of their classmates are the size and have the physical development of young adults. There is much variation.

Following our childhood and adolescent growth and development phase, we enter a darker, more variable phase of aging: deterioration and degeneration. Human deterioration is even more variable and less predictable than growth and development. Consider two 50-year-olds, for instance. One who is fit and youthful looking may appear to be 40 years old, while the other, who has lived a hard life, may appear to be 65 years old. If there is similar variation in older skeletons and comparable difficulties estimating their ages, then elderly skeletons may involve special problems for accurately estimating their ages. For a more detailed consideration of this problem, see Willey and Mann (1986).

An additional issue is the categories Bass et al (1971:160, table 40) used. Their oldest age category was greater than or equal to 50 years, and none of the skeletons was identified as being that old. The point of this discussion is that age estimations based on skeletons are limited and those limitations cause problems making reliable interpretations of the remains. Those inaccuracies have impacts on other studies, such as identifying and interpreting disease patterns, as we have syphilis.

Problems Identifying Disease in the Skeleton

Skeletal age estimation is only one of the challenges facing the osteologist. More directly affecting our mystery are the skeletal indications of illness. The skeleton has limited boney response to disease and injury.

Bone can only respond to stress and illness by increasing, decreasing, or both increasing and decreasing at the same time. That's all. An example of a disease that causes increase in bone is Paget's Disease, when many bones increase in thickness. An example of a bone-decreasing illness is osteoporosis, when bone walls become thinner and more susceptible to breaking. And an example of an illness with bone both increasing and decreasing is Pott's Disease, a manifestation of tuberculosis that involves vertebral body collapse (bone loss) while new bone forms around the collapsed vertebral body (bone increase). So, bones are limited in their response to

136

reflect the insults that diseases cause. They lack the expression variety and nuances that soft tissues often possess.

Complicating the limitation of bone response to illness, infected people may or may not manifest skeletal lesions. Disease manifestation depends on the characteristics of the disease, the person's fragility, and the environment. Take syphilis as an example. Take syphilis, please.

Just as some people infected with syphilis show variable soft tissue symptoms, only a small proportion of people who have untreated syphilis progressing to the tertiary phase show skeletal lesions from the disease. In an afflicted untreated group, as few as 1 percent (Gjestland 1955 in Ortner 2003: 279) and as high as 20 percent may have skeletal lesions (Resnick and Niwayama 1995 in Ortner 2003: 279). That means, conversely, that between 80 and 99 percent of tertiary syphilis victims show no diagnostic skeletal lesions at all.

How were these figures and assertions established? Much of what we know about untreated syphilis comes from three notorious studies (summarized by Powell and Cook 2005:23). In the US, the most infamous was the Tuskegee (Alabama) Syphilis Study (1932-1972) in which the course of the disease was followed in 431 untreated Black men. The study continued even after penicillin, the first effective treatment for the disease, became widely available. The second study was in Oslo (1890-1951), where 1,404 patients were denied standard treatment, researchers claiming that the treatment, which included the arsenic-based salvarsan, was more harmful than the normal course of the disease. Rosahn conducted the third study (1917-1947) using autopsy information from 382 US adults, some of whom were diagnosed with syphilis.

Leavenworth Site Skeletons and Syphilis

Now we have all of the figures needed to assess syphilis among the Leavenworth Site skeletons: namely, the number of Leavenworth adult skeletons, frequency of syphilis in an untreated population, and frequency of skeletal lesions in those individuals with tertiary syphilis. As established in the previous section, we assume that the rate of syphilis among the Leavenworth Arikara adults was between 5 and 10 percent. We further assume that of those Arikara adults with syphilis 1 to 20 percent displayed distinctive skeletal lesions. These figures are applied to the 100 Arikara adult skeletons from the Leavenworth Site and the resulting estimations are presented in Table 5.

The estimations indicate that only if a fairly high overall syphilis infection rate for the Leavenworth Arikara adults occurred and if a high skeletal lesion frequency also occurred, then—and only then—the expected number of identifiable syphilitic skeletons rises to a level that might produce a skeleton or two with diagnostic lesions. If lower, more conservative figures are employed, the probability of Leavenworth Site skeletal syphilis manifestations is low. So far we have only been dealing with acquired syphilis Acquired venereal syphilis is, of course, only one of the two forms of the disease.

In addition, we need to consider congenital venereal syphilis. Recall that no congenital syphilis markers were identified in the Leavenworth Site skeletons. There were no saddle-shaped faces, no saber shins, no mulberry molars, and no Hutchinson's incisors. But just as acquired syphilis' skeletal lesions may be ambiguous or absent, congenital syphilis' skeleton manifestations may be limited too.

The frequency of skeletal and dental alterations in congenital syphilis victims varies from study to study. In one study involving US adults (Fiumara and Lessell 1970 cited in Powell and Cook 2005: 47), 63% had Hutchinson's incisors, 65% had mulberry molars, and

Table 5. Expected number of Leavenworth Site skeletons having syphilitic lesions. Uses figure for adults (> 18 years individuals, n = 100) provided by Bass et al. (1971).

Frequency Showing Lesions	5% Syphilis Rate	10% Syphilis Rate
1%	0.05	0.1
5%	0.25	0.5
10%	0.5	1.0
15%	0.75	1.5
20%	1.0	2.0

73% had saddle-shaped noses. Some of these alterations would be visible in both subadults and adults.

There are complications, however, in calculating these rates for the Leavenworth Site Arikara skeletons. Susceptibility of the fetus to the spirochete differs depending on the fetus' developmental phase; it is most vulnerable in 2nd and 3rd trimesters. The other complication is the progress of the disease in the mother. Transmission of the spirochete from mother to fetus is highest in earlier phases of mother's infection (Stokes 1926 and 1944 in Powell and Cook 2005:24). It is difficult to estimate how many of the Leavenworth Site skeletons might show the effects of congenital syphilis. For that estimation we need to know the probability that a pregnant female was infected with syphilis and in the early stages of the disease, and that her fetus was in the 2nd or 3rd trimesters. These variables are too complicated to address here.

To summarize, the skeleton has much to tell about its previous occupant, but it is also ambiguous on many points. The skeleton may not permit accurate age estimations (especially for elderly adults) or allow definitive disease identifications. Despite these limitations, if syphilis was persistent and prevalent among the Leavenworth Site Arikara, we would expect at least a few skeletons and teeth to indicate the disease's presence. None were reported from the Leaven-worth Site.

Change in Syphilitic Manifestations

Microbes, as all living organisms, are not static immutable entities. They change, adapt and evolve. And as the microbes change, their expression and manifestations on their hosts may change as well. In addition to the microbes, the host adapts and evolves to the microbe's assault. As a consequence of this parry-and-foil sequence, co-evolution occurs, encompassing adaptations of both pathogen and host to one another.

Using co-evolution as a foundation, we consider whether the causative agent of syphilis, the bacterium *Treponema pallidum*, has changed. If the spirochete has changed, then the manifestations of syphilis in the early 1800s may not be the same as those of the early 1900s, when most of the studies of untreated victims were conducted. Some infectious diseases are highly adaptable, capable of changing quickly to surmount the host's defense mechanisms.

Tuberculosis is one of these malleable diseases that can change quickly. It is an illness caused by *Mycobacterium tuberculosis*, which usually attacks the lungs, although other organs can be involved. During the 19th century, the US experienced severe effects of the disease. "Consumption," as it was commonly known then, was the greatest year-to-year killer. It targeted those people living in crowded conditions and members of other vulnerable groups, including the poor and destitute. Arikara, for instance, were adversely affected by the disease during the 19th century.

By the mid-19th century, however, progress against the tuberculosis was underway. R. Koch identified the microorganism responsible for the disease in 1882, thus leading to a means of identifying its victims—whether they were symptomatic or not. There were also improvements in the standard of living: better nutrition and better housing as well as isolation of the disease's victims in sanatoriums.

Treatments of the disease had varying efficacy. By the 1950s, following the development of antibiotics, particularly steptomycium, tuberculosis was well under control, if not virtually eliminated in the West. With time and adapting generations of *Mycobacterium tuberculosis*, however, the organism developed genetic defenses to antibiotics and resistance to their effectiveness.

With this adaptation by the tuberculosis microbe, dosages of previously effective drugs became ineffective. Some tuberculosis strains, for instance, became resistant to streptomycin. By the mid-1980s and into the early 1990s, there were annual increases in the incidence of and mortality from the disease in the US. Currently a combination, a "cocktail," of four antibiotics is used to treat the disease, which adapted and became resistant to solitary drugs. Tuberculosis is an example of a rapidly changing disease.

Could the organism causing venereal syphilis change as rapidly as tuberculosis? Could 19th century syphilis be less virulent than the 20th century form? That does not seem to be the case.

The causative agent of venereal syphilis, *Treponema pallidum*, shows no such quick adaptations. The spirochete is effectively treated, at least in the early stages of the disease, by courses of penicillin or other antibiotics. All indications suggest that the syphilis spirochete is as vulnerable to treatment with penicillin now as it was 60 years ago when the drug was first developed (reviewed in Powell and Cook 2005:10-11). The disease agent is relatively stable and we suspect that the skeletal alterations of the disease are likewise stable. So syphilis seems relatively stable, at least contrasted with some other infectious agents, such as tuberculosis. Based on this conclusion, the 19th century skeletal manifestations of syphilis were probably the same as the 20th century ones.

Summary

There are five biological explanations we have considered to explain the mystery of the bones. It is possible that the osteological conclusions are incorrect; these errors could have been caused by poor skeletal and dental preservation or misinterpretations of the disease manifestations. Secondly, it is possible that the Arikara had developed genetic resistance to syphilis; perhaps blood type O is better adapted to combating the disease. Thirdly, it is possible that the 19th century Arikara were too short-lived to manifest the skeletal defects associated with tertiary syphilis. Fourthly, it is possible that the limited nature of skeletal response to disease failed to reflect diagnostic indications of syphilis. And finally it is possible that syphilis and its manifestations changed in the century between occupation of the Leavenworth Site and when studies documented the impact of syphilis on the skeleton. These biological explanations are discussed in the next chapter.

8. Discussion

In previous chapters, we presented what members of the Lewis and Clark Expedition wrote concerning the Arikara and assessed their observations. Some researchers take these descriptions of their voyage verbatim, as Gospel. Employing this perspective, the empirical universe is rearranged to fit descriptions of events expedition members recorded during their four-year journey. Without critically assessing the "Book of Lewis and Clark," however, they suffer the deception of all true believers. "Lewis and Clark wrote it, we believe it, and that's enough!" They, in brief, become a cult. In this book, we have tried to avoid that fate.

There are several final issues we need to address to complete our assessment of the historical accounts and the Arikara bones. First we present a discussion involving the ramifications that our study has for the debate concerning the New World or Old World origin of syphilis. Next we consider the reburial issue and how it impacts our approach to understanding the past. And finally we evaluate our assumption that the disease the Arikara had was syphilis. After discussing these three topics, we present the summary and conclusions in the final chapter.

PreColumbian or Columbian Origin of Syphilis?

Our study has implications for the question of the New World vs. Old World origin of venereal syphilis. That debate goes like this. Was syphilis a New World disease, carried by Columbus or his crewmembers returning to Europe in 1493 or perhaps on one of their subsequent trips? According to this view, syphilis was carried to Europe by returning crewmembers, became established there, and from Europe spread across Asia and Africa in a matter of a few decades.

The alternate view, in contrast, claims syphilis was an Old World disease. According to this view, syphilis was present in the Old World long before Columbus' voyages. But syphilis was only diagnostically recognized about 1500AD, coincidentally with European discovery of the Americas. And it was this diagnosis—a medical identification, not the disease—that spread across the Old World in a few decades.

This debate has a long history, persisting for the past 500 years. What do the 19th century Arikara bones say about this issue?

Before showing how our mystery applies to this grand debate, there are some assumptions required. Let's assume that the historical accounts and our interpretations of them are correct: syphilis was present among the 19th century Arikara. And let's also assume that none of the Leavenworth Site skeletons show signs of the disease. After all, there are none of the classic skeletal indicators of syphilis. We have argued both these points throughout this work.

If those assumptions are correct, syphilis may have been present in the PreColumbian Americas. And whatever explains the absence of syphilis in 19th century Arikara skeletons— biological adaptations to the disease, limitations of the skeletal system, limitations of the archaeological and osteological records, etc.—may also explain the absence of syphilis in other PreColumbian American skeletons. According to this proposal, here is a uniform explanation for the absence of syphilis lesion in both the PreColumbian and early 19th century Arikara.

Assuming syphilis was present in 19th century Arikara—as Lewis and Clark and others seem to claim—and there is no skeletal evidence of its presence, then we should not expect other skeletal series to show the disease either. That conclusion applies whatever the time period, whether the skeletal collections are from the historic or prehistoric time period. By extension based on the 19th century Arikara case, we expect little skeletal evidence for syphilis in the New World even if it was endemic in the Americas during PreColumbian times. That absence is consistent with what prehistoric American remains indicate. In this respect, our results are consistent with Cook and Powell's (2005) conservative assessment in their Pan-American summary of syphilis. They found no definitive skeletal indications of widespread PreColumbian syphilis in the Americas, although some form of treponematosis was present. But of course the absence of skeletal indications of syphilis does not prove its presence. So this explanation requires further testing before it is accepted.

Native American Graves and Repatriation Act

We are fortunate to have had access to information about Arikara bones from the Leavenworth Site cemeteries that Bass excavated in the 1960s. Without his dogged fieldwork and cemetery excavations, the questions we have raised could not have been addressed. Unfortunately, today comparable archaeological recovery of Native American remains is impossible, as it has been for the past two decades.

There is one matter that has had a tremendous impact on how we study and understand the past, including questions such as those we have addressed here. That issue is repatriation of Native American skeletal remains and objects of cultural patrimony. The Native American Graves and Repatriation Act (NAGPRA), which was enacted in 1990, requires inventory of Native American skeletons and artifacts of cultural patrimony, notification of the most likely descendants, and at their request, delivery of bones and artifacts to them. Museums, colleges and other institutions that hold collections of Native American human remains and sensitive artifacts are required to initiate the process.

The first response by the scientific community was predictably negative. Our understanding and interpretation of the past, they cried, would be permanently altered. Subsequent assessments by some scientists were more positive—the equivalent of "sweet" grapes instead of sour grapes. These positivists saw NAGPRA eliminating gaps in temporal and geographic data as skeletal collections were analyzed in preparation for repatriation. They anticipated inventory and analysis of remains occurring as funding for such studies increased. Even better, those analyses were to be performed in a more systematic and detailed fashion than previous attempts had provided. And these efforts, while increasing knowledge about the past, would also result in more ethical dealings with Native Americans (Rose et al. 1996, Klesert and Powell 1993). They foresaw, as one article put it, a "vibrant future for North American osteology" (Rose et al. 1996:81).

However laudable such a law may be, NAGPRA raises as many questions as it settles. Many of those complications have come forth and been focused with the discovery of ancient Kennewick man.

Eight years after NAGPRA was enacted, a human skeleton was discovered eroding from the banks of the Columbia River near Kennewick, Washington. Processed as a forensic case, the initial assessment was the skeleton was that of a 40-50 year-old, medium-tall male of Caucasoid heritage. Inconsistent with a recent death, however, an ancient projectile point was embedded in the innominate, a point that usually dates 4500 to 9000 years. Radiocarbon dating of bone supported an even earlier date: about 9500 BP. The Corps of Engineers, who oversees that section of the Columbia River, determined that the Kennewick skeleton should be delivered to Native American groups of that region led by the Confederated Tribes of the Umatilla Indian Reservation. Scientists objected, claiming that Kennewick's Caucasoid features contradicted its cultural affiliation with the Umatilla, or any other Native Americans for that matter. And with that opposition, the question of possession and control of the remains went careening through the legal system (Thomas 2000, Powell 2005). In 2004, a US Court of Appeals decision indicated that Kennewick was so ancient that it was not Native American, at least as defined by NAGPRA, and that scientific analysis of the remains could proceed (http://www.ca9.uscourts.gov/ca9/newopinions.nsf/AAFB80F54839DD2D8 8256E300069CF95/$file/0235994.pdf?openelement, accessed June 30, 2007).

The final, deciding issue was—and still is—one of heritage. Who are the descendants of Kennewick? What group is the closest descendant group? Whoever it might be, biological evidence indicates it was not the Umatilla.

Contrasted with the Kennewick situation, there is little doubt that the Leavenworth Site skeletons were Arikara. That determination is based on historic accounts as well as archaeological and osteological evidence. Some of the skeletons from the Leavenworth Site have undergone analysis anticipating repatriation, and have already been returned and reburied. In the 1980s, the W.H. Over collection was returned to a pan-tribal organization and those several skeletons were reburied. The 37 Leavenworth Site skeletons excavated by Stirling and Strong for the Smithsonian Institution have been inventoried; negotiations with the Arikara are underway, and they are being prepared for transferal to the Three Affiliated Tribes for reburial. The Bass collection from the Leavenworth Site, the 285 skeletons employed in this work, was inventoried, the Arikara notified, and the remains' return have not been requested so they are still curated at the University of Tennessee—Knoxville (Lee Meadows Jantz, personal communication).

As these collections are buried, new questions will be difficult to address. How we study the past and understand it has been changed—for better and worse—by repatriation.

As an example of this change, Weiss (2006:1) found that following NAGPRA's enactment, studies of skeletal biology of Native American remains in the major US physical anthropology journal plummeted. The number of articles in the national journal of physical anthropology was compared before and after the enactment of NAGPRA. There were a smaller percentage of articles dealing with Native American skeletal remains. In addition, following enactment of NAGPRA, fewer sites and fewer geographic locations were presented in those articles. Rather than increasing knowledge, as some positivists claimed, this first assessment of NAGPRA's impact indicates the reverse (Weiss 2006).

So, based on these preliminary results from a national journal, there is a decrease in the study of Native American skeletons following NAGPRA's enactment—as might have been predicted. The optimism of earlier predictions (Rose et al. 1996, Klesert and Powell 1993) is not founded based on these results. And future osteological excavations and studies will be limited by what has been anticipated and performed in the past.

148

Venereal Disease Other than Syphilis

There is a critical question that needs to be raised, one that was only tangentially addressed earlier in our presentation. Throughout this work, we have argued that the venereal disease the 19th century Arikara had was syphilis, the disease most consistent with the historic accounts and dates the symptoms appeared.

But what if the disease expedition members suffered and Lewis and Clark described was not syphilis, as we have argued here? What if the disease was gonorrhea or some other sexually transmitted disease? The skeletal markers of gonorrhea and the other venereal diseases are not nearly so definitive or identifiable as those of syphilis and those skeletal alterations might easily be misidentified by osteologists as some other ailments—if noticed at all.

So, if the Arikara's disease that was described in the historic documents is something other than syphilis, the skeletal indicators of that other disease become difficult to discern and the probability of definitive skeletal manifestations among the Leavenworth skeletons declines. There is the possibility, then, that throughout this tome we have misrepresented the issue and a major assumption of our thesis is in error. The probability of this possibility is uncertain, although we consider it unlikely.

We consider such an error unlikely for two reasons. The timing of the expedition members' venereal symptoms coincides best with syphilis. Had the disease been one other than syphilis, a different sequence of symptoms would have occurred rather than those recorded. The second reason such an error is unlikely is that a trained physician identified syphilis was among the Arikara later in the century. Although that physician's identification occurred five decades after Lewis and Clark's Arikara visit, the persistence of syphilis in a population would be expected, at least until effective treatments were developed in the following century.

Summary

There are three issues presented in this discussion. First, there is the possibility of syphilis being present in the Americas before Columbus' voyages and the implications of the early 19th century Arikara skeletons. If the 19th century Arikara skeletons had syphilis—as we have argued, but the 300 Arikara skeletons do not show any skeletal indications of the disease—as we have also argued, then we would similarly not expect syphilis-infected PreColumbian skeletons to show indications of the disease.

Second, NAGPRA has altered our way of interpreting the past. The initial impact has been stifling, the ultimate effect over the next few decades may prove devastating both for Native Americans and rational people worldwide. Ours is but a small and relatively successful story in this epic loss.

Third, we have deduced that the disease present among the Arikara was syphilis. The diagnosis and incubation time the historic accounts report are consistent with syphilis, and syphilis is the most likely venereal disease. But what if the disease reported was another one other than syphilis? If that is the case—if the disease is not syphilis—then our conclusions need to be reassessed and the whole issue reevaluated.

9. Summary and Conclusions

During Lewis and Clark's epic journey, they noted previously undescribed places, undocumented plants, extraordinary animals, and uncharted rivers. Among their observations, they described the peoples they met, peoples who were thoroughly familiar with the places, plants, animals, and rivers that amazed the explorers as they later did the outside world.

Among the many native groups the expedition encountered, they visited the Arikara, who were then living in three villages on the Missouri River near the mouth of the Grand River. There they treated and counseled with the Arikara, staying for a few days.

Brief as their stay was, it was time enough for sexual encounters between expedition members and Arikara. Some of those encounters were mentioned in their accounts. Clark's writings best document the associations. And if there is any doubt about sexual encounters between expedition members and Arikara, disease symptoms occurred in the incubation period expected of syphilis.

The expedition's chroniclers are not the only ones who noted the Arikara women's sexual availability and the resulting venereal infections. Several other late 18th and early 19th century travelers and traders made similar observations.

Two of the three Arikara villages that Lewis and Clark visited in the early 19th century were archaeologically excavated in the 20th century. And those archaeological excavations included parts of the associated cemeteries. Recovered Arikara skeletons were analyzed and reported, and those several hundred studied skeletons showed no indications of syphilis. This is the mystery we have sought to explain.

We presented a number of possible explanations for the apparent discrepancy between the historic accounts of the Arikara possessing venereal disease and the bones from the Leavenworth Site lacking such lesions. Those explanations were divided into historic and behavioral explanations on the one hand, and biological and evolutionary approaches on the other hand. Before reviewing those explanations, however, we presented the chroniclers' accounts and osteologists' conclusions

Historic Accounts

Our first approach to evaluate the historical documents compared Lewis and Clark's observations with those of others who saw the Arikara in the late 18th and early 19th centuries. It behooves us to evaluate Lewis and Clark's accounts—as all forms of evidence—with a cautious eye to see what is reasonable, what is feasible, and what is not. For our purposes, the issues of Arikara sexual availability and the presence of venereal disease among the Arikara were the key points of interest.

For the most part, contemporary observers supported and elaborated Lewis and Clark's accounts. Concerning the sexual availability of the Arikara women, Trudeau, Tabeau, Bradbury, Brackenridge, and Luttig all concurred with Lewis and Clark: the Arikara were sexually active and available to white traders and travelers. There was consensus, too, concerning venereal disease. As Lewis and Clark, other observers—including Trudeau, Tabeau, Bradbury and Brackenridge, Denig, and Hayden—noted venereal disease or venereal diseases among the Arikara. They either observed the illness directly among the Arikara or as the result of party members' sexual encounters with Arikara. So, there was agreement among most historic documents that the Arikara women were sexually available, at least to some white transients in some contexts, and that venereal disease was present among them and transmitted to some of their white partners.

Where there were discrepancies between the accounts, these differences tended to involve issues of lesser importance to our discussion. One of those contentious issues concerned the "depravity" of the Arikara women. From what Lewis and Clark as well as Tabeau and several other travelers wrote, there seemed to be few—if any—"virtuous" 19th century Arikara women. However Brackenridge's account of a public ceremony in the Arikara village that rewarded female chastity, and Luttig's account of an Arikara woman visiting his trading post desiring marriage, not sex for hire, showed complexity in the issue. These accounts indicated that at least some Arikara women in at least some situations were not the common chattel that other observers would have had us believe. Unfortunately, the reasons and cultural contexts for these situations were not mentioned in the accounts and those social circumstances remain unclear today. There were a few other contrasts within the historic accounts.

Another issue where the historic accounts differed among themselves is whether the venereal disease present among the Arikara was treatable or not. Lewis and Clark omitted mention of native treatments for venereal disease. They had more than enough to do during their brief Arikara visit, and besides, they carried their own venereal disease medicines and treatments based on principles of western medicine. Tabeau argued that venereal disease was not treated. Trudeau and Bradbury, on the contrary, indicated the reverse. They claimed the venereal disease was thoroughly treatable with common plants and well-known remedies.

Along a similar vein concerning infectious virulence, Tabeau described the venereal disease as being strong and invasive among the Arikara—as implied from Clark's account, while Bradbury indicated the opposite. Bradbury claimed it was a mild and benign form of the illness.

A final dispute among the chroniclers was the beauty of the Arikara women. Gass and Brackenridge found them attractive— perhaps very attractive, if you know what we mean. Tabeau, so often the naysayer in other issues, had nothing good to write about the beauty of Arikara women. From his writings, they all seemed to be ugly hags.

Many of these historic accounts denigrate and demean the Arikara. Is it possible that there was a concerted effort to misrepresent the truth and debase the Arikara? Such a conspiracy on the part of so many, relatively independent travelers and traders seemed unlikely.

Arikara Skeletons

To assess the accuracy of historical observations, we employed a different information source concerning the early 19th century Arikara other than the written documents. This alternate source of information, the Arikara skeletons, was tangible and had the hardness of bone—literally the durability, but also the mutability of bone.

We presented descriptions of the skeletons archaeologically recovered from the villages where Lewis and Clark visited the Arikara, now called the Leavenworth Site. The way we figured it, if the historic accounts of Lewis and Clark and others accurately depicted Arikara sexual license and presence of venereal disease, as they appeared to do, the Arikara skeletons should have shown the ravages of venereal disease. But they did not. Three hundred Leavenworth Site skeletons showed none of the classic signs of syphilis: no caries sicca, no saber shins, no mulberry molars, and no Hutchinson's incisors.

How do we explain the discrepancy between the absence of syphilitic lesions among the skeletons from the Leavenworth Site and the contrasting historic accounts? Which—if either—is correct? To answer those questions, we considered historic explanations and biological explanations.

Historic and Ethnographic Explanations

We first turned to the historic documents and ethnographic accounts for answers. In an earlier section of this summary, we evaluated the historic accounts, finding them consistent on many matters. That leaves two additional historic and ethnographic issues to review. Did the 19th century Arikara have effective traditional treatments for venereal disease? Or did the 19th century Arikara have syphilis and its telling tertiary stigmata and choose to bury the afflicted elsewhere other than the cemeteries close-by the villages?

A possible explanation for this mystery was that the 19th century Arikara had effective means of treating venereal disease. This claim was in keeping with Bradbury and Trudeau's historical accounts. Most often identified among these medicinal lines, indigenous plants were mentioned to treat illness. The plant that attracted the most attention in the 19th and early 20th century accounts was purple coneflower (most likely *Echinacea angustifolia*). Bradbury noted its roots being used by his afflicted party members, and the plant was embraced by later herbalists to treat syphilis, as well as many other ailments. As far as we can discern, however, the first truly effective syphilis treatment was penicillin, which became available in the mid-1940s, nearly a century and a half after Lewis and Clark's journey. So, unless an effective herbal cure was known in the 19th century and its efficacy ignored by mainstream medicine, an effective ethnopharmaceutical cure seems unlikely.

There was another cultural and historic explanation for the human bone vs. written account discrepancy. That explanation involved different mortuary treatment for the afflicted.

Archaeologists recovered only a small portion of the deaths the Arikara must have suffered while residing at the Leavenworth Site. Based on the number of skeletons estimated to be at the Leavenworth Site (350 to 400 skeletons) and number of years the villages were occupied (about 28 years), the average deaths per year numbered only 12.5 to 14.3. This average number of deaths is remarkably low for the villages whose populations were estimated to be at least 2,000 people. If a normal death rate is assumed and all deaths were buried in the cemeteries adjacent to the villages, then the number of recovered skeletons was only 10 percent of those expected to have been present. Therefore, 90 percent of the skeletons were not archaeologically recovered.

It is possible that there were special locations or special mortuary handling of unusual or "different" individuals. And those Arikara displaying the effects of tertiary syphilis certainly would have been different. It is possible, this explanation claims, that syphilis was present among the Arikara, and that a proportion of those afflicted developed and showed tertiary skeletal stigmata. But the affected corpses, which were considered "ritually unclean" in the eyes of the Arikara, were buried in locations other than the usual Arikara cemeteries. And it was the usual cemeteries that archaeologists excavated in the 1900s, not the extraordinary ones. As an analogy to those Arikara who may have died displaying carries sicca, we presented the tale concerning the plight of the scalped Arikara man. Surviving his scalping, he then lived a solitary, furtive life, and when he died, was excluded from normal cemetery burial. Perhaps a similar isolated burial befell the early 19th century Arikara who manifested the stigmata of tertiary syphilis.

Skeletal and Biological Explanations

The historic and ethnographic accounts and cultural explanations are not alone in their ambiguity. In addition to possible historic and ethnographic explanations, there are several explanations involving skeletal and biological processes. It is obvious that the archaeological record is biased, as are the historic accounts. Archaeology is limited to inferences made from materials that persist and preserve over the centuries, and that can be found and recovered for study. And for our purposes, we presume that the presence of disease can be correctly identified and accurately interpreted.

There were four biological explanations we explored to explain the mystery. First, Arikara, as many other Native Americans, may have had genetic resistance to syphilis. Support for this explanation came from early 20th century research on blood types and syphilis recovery successes. Individuals with blood type O recovered more readily and were less likely to show skeletal lesions associated with syphilis than those with the other blood types. And most Native Americans, presumably including early 19th century Arikara, were blood type O, thus more resistant to syphilis.

Second, it was possible that the 19th century Arikara were too short-lived to manifest the tertiary skeletal indications of syphilis. Their lives were so short and the effects of syphilis so slow, this explanation claimed, that Arikara bones were not altered by the tertiary phase of the disease.

Third, it was possible that the osteological assessments concerning the absence of syphilis were wrong. Contributing to these osteological errors may have been some bones' and teeth poor preservation, osteologists' misidentification of diseases present, and traditional Arikara cultural practices—such as dental attrition, for instance.

And the final biological explanation claimed that syphilis changed in the past 200 years. It was possible that 19th century syphilis changed so much that by the 20th century our expectations of the syphilis's manifestations, based on evidence from the more recent forms of the disease, misrepresented the earlier form of the disease.

Conclusions

Early white travelers who ascended the Missouri River noted both the sexual availability of Native American women and the prevalence of syphilis.

Syphilis can be manifest in the bones. Children born with syphilis tend to have notched screw-driver-shaped incisor teeth, bowed shinbones and sunken noses. Adults with long-term syphilis can have eroded areas of the skull, erosion that leaves the bones looking worm-eaten, as well as bowed shins.

The Lewis and Clark Expedition members, as other travelers, noted the availability of women, especially among the Arikara, and the presence of venereal disease. The Arikara left large cemeteries. The bones buried there have been collected by two generations of archaeologists and studied by several generations of osteologists. These bones should show syphilitic lesions. But they do not. How can we explain this mystery?

Our attempt to unravel this puzzle has examined many factors. Could all the early explorers have been wrong in their assessment of the disease? Were the Arikara able to treat their infections, thus reducing or eliminating bone damage? And what of the carefully examined bones? Did the Arikara bury their syphilitic members somewhere other than the community cemeteries? Did the Indians live such short lives that there was not enough time to develop the bone changes? Has the biology of the syphilis spirochete changed in two centuries?

In conducting that quest, we used as many avenues as possible to determine the truth concerning the past. From these multiple sources, we determined what is reasonable from the historical accounts using measured conclusions from archaeology and osteology. Employing sources from humanities, social sciences and biological sciences helped us interpret the past.

We have examined many possibilities and laid out the facts. The reader is invited to join us in the quest for understanding—the Mystery of the Bones.

References Cited

Abel, Annie Heloise (Editor)
1932. *Chardon's Journal at Fort Clark 1834-1839*. State of South Dakota, Department of History, Pierre.

_____

1939. *Tabeau's Narrative of Loisel's Expedition to the Upper Missouri*. University of Oklahoma Press, Norman.

Aufderheide, Arthur C., and Conrado Rodriguez-Martin
1998. *The Cambridge Encyclopedia of Human Paleopathology*. Cambridge University Press, Cambridge.

Bass, William M., David R. Evans, and Richard L. Jantz
1971. The Leavenworth Site Cemetery: Archaeology and Physical Anthropology. *University of Kansas Publications in Anthropology,* no. 2.

Bass, William M., and Terrell W. Phenice
1975. Prehistoric Human Skeletal Material from Three Sites in North and South Dakota. Appendix C in Robert W. Neuman The Sonota Complex and Associated Sites on the Northern Plains, Nebraska State Historical Society *Publications in Anthropology* 6:106-140

Biddle, Nicholas
1814. *History of the Expedition under the Command of Captains Lewis and Clark*. Bradford and Inskeep, Philadelphia. (Reprinted 1966 University Microfilms, Ann Arbor, IL.)

Blakeslee, Donald J.
1981. Toward a Cultural Understanding of Human Microevolution on the Great Plains. IN R.L. Jantz and D.H. Ubelaker (eds.) Progress in Skeletal Biology of Plains Populations, *Plains Anthropologist Memoir* 17 (vol. 26, no. 94, pt. 2), pp. 93-106.

Blankinship, J.W.
1905. Native Economic Plants of Montana. Montana Agricultural College Experimental Station, Bulletin 56.

Brackenridge, H.M.
1906. Journal of a Voyage up the River Missouri; Performed in Eighteen Hundred and Eleven. 2nd edition. IN Reuben Gold Thwaites (ed.) *Early Western Travels*, vol. 6, pp.21-166. (Reprinted by AMS Press, New York, 1966.)

Bradbury, John
1904. Travels in the Interior of America in the Years 1809, 1810, and 1811. 2nd edition. IN Reuben Gold Thwaites (ed.) *Early Western Travels*, vol. 5. (Reprinted by AMS Press, New York, 1966.)

Chuinard, E.G.
1979. *Only One Man Died: The Medical Aspects of the Lewis and Clark Expedition*. A.H. Clark, Glendale, CA.

Cook, Della Collins, and Mary Lucas Powell
2005. Piecing the Puzzle Together: North American Treponematosis Overview. IN M.L. Powell and D.C. Cook (eds.) *The Myth of Syphilis*, University Press of Florida, Gainesville. Pages 442-479.

Cutright, Paul R.
1969. *Lewis and Clark: Pioneering Naturalists*. University of Illinois Press, Urbana.

Curtis, Edward S.
1907-1930. *The North American Indian*. The University Press, Cambridge. (Reprinted 1970 by Johnson Reprint Corp., New York, NY.)

DeMaille, Raymond J.
2001. Introduction. IN R.J. DeMaille (ed.) *Handbook of North American Indians: Plains*, vol. 13, pt. 1, pp. 1-13. Smithsonian Institution Press, Washington, DC.

Denig, Edwin Thompson
1961. *Five Indian Tribes of the Upper Missouri: Sioux, Arickaras, Assiniboines, Crees, Crows.* University of Oklahoma Press, Norman.

Drumm, Stella (Editor)
1920. *Journal of a Fur-trading Expedition on the Upper Missouri, 1812-1813.* Argosy-Antiquarian Limited, New York. (1964 edition).

Duke, Jones A.
2002. *Handbook of Medicinal Herbs.* CRC Press, Boca Raton, FL.

Durkee, Silas
1866 . *A Treatise on Gonorrhoea and Syphilis.* J.P. Jewett and Co., Boston.

Ewers, John C.
1961. Editor's Introduction. IN E.T. Denig's *Five Indian Tribes of the Upper Missouri*, University of Oklahoma Press, pp. xiii-xxxvii.

———
1968. *Indian Life on the Upper Missouri.* University of Oklahoma Press, Norman.

Fenner, F., D.A. Henderson, I. Arita, Z. Jezek, and I.D. Ladnyi
1988. *Smallpox and Its Eradication.* World Health Organization, Geneva.

Foster, Steven
1985. Echinacea Exalted! 2nd edition. Ozark Beneficial Plant Project, Brixley, MO.

Gjestland, T.
1955. *The Oslo Study of Untreated Syphilis.* Akademisk Forlag, Oslo.

Gilman, Sander L.
1988. *Diseases and Representation: Images of Illness from Madness to AIDS.* Cornell University Press, Ithaca.

Gilmore, Melvin R.
1991 . *Uses of Plants by the Indians of the Missouri River Region.* University of Nebraska Press, Lincoln.

Goff, C.W.
1967. Syphilis. IN D. Brothwell and A.T. Sandison (eds.) *Diseases in Antiquity*, C.C. Thomas, Springfield, IL. Pages 279-294.

Gray, Margery P., and William M. Laughlin
1960. Blood Groups of Caddoan Indians in Oklahoma. *American Journal of Human Genetics* 12:86-94.

Great Plains Flora Association
1986. *Flora of the Great Plains.* University Press of Kansas, Lawrence.

Gregg, John B., and Pauline S. Gregg
1987. *Dry Bones: Dakota Territory Reflected.* Sioux Printing, Sioux Falls, SD.

Hamperl, H.
1967. The Osteological Consequences of Scalping. IN D. Brothwell and A.T. Sandison (eds.) *Diseases in Antiquity*, C.C. Thomas, Springfield, IL. Pages 630-634.

Hamperl, H., and W.S. Laughlin
1959. Osteological Consequences of Scalping. *Human Biology* 31: 80-89.

Hart, Jeff
1992. *Montana Native Plants and Early Peoples.* Montana Historical Society Press, Helena.

Hayden, F.V.
1862. On the Ethnography and Philology of the Indian Tribes of the Missouri Valley. *Transactions of the American Philosophical Society* 12 (Art. 3): 231-464.

Hodges, Denise C., and Shirley J. Shermer
2005. Treponematosis in the Northern and Central Great Plains. IN M.L. Powell and D.C. Cook (eds.) *The Myth of Syphilis: The Natural History of Treponematosis in North America,* University Press of Florida, Gainesville. Pages 200-226.

Holder, Preston
1970. *The Hoe and the Horse on the Plains: A Study of Cultural Development among North American Indians.* University of Nebraska Press, Lincoln.

Hollimon, Sandra E., and Douglas W. Owsley
1994. Osteology of the Fay Tolton Site: Implications for Warfare during the Intial Middle Missouri Variant. IN D.W. Owsley and R.L. Jantz (eds.) *Biology in the Great Plains: Migration, Warfare, Health, and Subsistence,* Smithsonian Institution Press, Washington. Pages 345-353.

Jackson, Donald D. (Editor)
1978. *Letters of the Lewis and Clark Expedition with Related Documents.* University of Illinois Press, Urbana. 2 volumes.

James, Edwin
1966. Account of an Expedition from Pittsburgh to the Rocky Mountains. IN Reuben Gold Thwaites (ed.) *Early Western Travels,* vol. 14. (Reprinted AMS Press, New York.)

Johnston, Alex
1987. *Plants and the Blackfoot.* Lethbridge Historical Society, Lethbridge, Alberta.

Kindscher, Kelly
1992 . *Medicinal Wild Plants of the Prairie: An Ethnobotanical Guide.* University of Kansas, Lawrence.

Klesert, Anthony L., and Shirley Powell
1993. A Perspective on Ethics and the Reburial Controversy. *American Antiquity* 58: 348-354.

Krause, Richard A.
1972. The Leavenworth Site: Archaeology of an Historic Arikara Community. *University of Kansas Publications in Anthropology,* no. 3.

Lowry, Thomas P.
2004. *Venereal Disease and the Lewis and Clark Expedition.* University of Nebraska Press, Lincoln.

Lowry, Thomas P., and P. Willey
2007. The Mystery of the Bones. *We Proceeded On* 33(1):22-26.

Luttig, John C. (Stella M. Drumm, editor)
1964. *Journal of a Fur-Trading Expedition on the Upper Missouri, 1812-1813.* Argosy-Antiquarian Limited, New York.

McElligott, G.
1960 . Venereal Disease and the Public Health. *Journal of Venereal Diseases* 36:207-215.

Merbs, Charles F.
1992. A New World of Infectious Disease. *Yearbook of Physical Anthropology* 35:3-42.

Michelson, Truman
1932. The Narrative of a Southern Cheyenne Woman. *Smithsonian Miscellaneous Collections* 87(5):1-13.

Morgan, Dale L.
1953. *Jedediah Smith and the Opening of the West.* University of Nebraska Press, Lincoln.

Moulton, Gary E. (Editor)
2002-2004. *The Definitive Journals of Lewis and Clark.* Bison Books, Lincoln, Nebraska.

Murphy, Lawrence R.
1985. The Enemy among Us: Venereal Disease among Union Soldiers in the Far West. *Civil War History* 31 (3):257.

Ordway, John (Milo M. Quaife, editor)
1916. The Journals of Captain Meriwether Lewis and Sergeant John Ordway Kept on the Expedition of Western Exploration, 1803-1806. *Collections of the State Historical Society of Wisconsin* vol. 22. (Second printing 1965, Cushing-Malloy, Inc., Ann Arbor.)

Ortner, Donald J.
2003. *Identification of Pathological Conditions in Human Skeletal Remains.* 2nd edition. Academic Press, Amsterdam.

Ortner, Donald J., and Walter G.J. Putschar
1985. Identification of Pathological Conditions in Human Skeletal Remains. *Smithsonian Contributions to Anthropology*, no. 28. Reprint edition.

Osler, William.
1893. *The Principles and Practice of Medicine.* Appleton and Company, NY.

Owlsey, Douglas W.
1992. Demography of Prehistoric and Early Historic Northern Plains Populations. IN J.W. Verano and D.H. Ubelaker (eds.) *Disease and Demography in the Americas*, Smithsonian Institution Press, Washington, DC. Pages 75-86.

Owsley, Douglas W., and Richard L. Jantz
1994. An Interpretative Approach to Great Plains Skeletal Biology. IN D.W. Owsley and R.L. Jantz (editors) *Skeletal Biology in the Great Plains*, Smithsonian Institution Press, Washington, DC. Pages 3-8.

Palkovich, Ann M.
1981. Demography and Disease Patterns in a Protohistoric Plains Group: A Study of the Mobridge Site (39WW1). *Plains Anthropologist Memoir* 17 (26-94, pt. 2): 71-84.

Parks, Douglas R.
1982. An Historical Character Mythologized: The Scalped Man in Arikara and Pawnee Folklore. IN D.H. Ubelaker and H.J. Viola (eds.) Plains Indian Studies: A Collection of Essays in Honor of John C. Ewers and Waldo R. Wedel. *Smithsonian Contributions to Anthropology*, no. 30: 47-58.

2001. Arikara. IN R.J. DeMaille (ed.) *Handbook of North American Indians: Plains*, vol. 13, pp. 365-390. Smithsonian Institution Press, Washington, DC.

Powell, Joseph F.
2005. *The First American: Race, Evolution, and the Origin of Native Americans*. Cambridge University Press, Cambridge.

Powell, Mary Lucas, and Della Collins Cook
2005. Treponematosis. IN M.L. Powell and D.C. Cook (eds.) *The Myth of Syphilis: The Natural History of Treponematosis in North America*, University Press of Florida, Gainesville. Pages 9-62.

Powers, Marla
1986. *Oglala Women*. University of Chicago Press, Chicago.

Pratt, David
1999. Lessons for Implementation from the World's Most Successful Programme: The Global Eradication of Smallpox. *Journal of Curriculum Studies* 2:177-194.

Resnick, D. and G. Niwayama
1995. Osteomyelitis, Septic Arthritis, and Soft Tissue Infection: Organisms. IN D. Resnick (ed.) *Diagnosis of Bone and Joint Disorders*, 3rd edition, Saunders, Philadelphia. Pages 2448-2558.

Rickett, H.W.
1950. John Bradbury's Explorations in Missouri Territory. *Proceedings of the American Philosophical Society* 94:59-89.

Ronda, James P.
1984. *Lewis and Clark among the Indians*. University of Nebraska Press, Lincoln.

Rose, Jerome C., Thomas J. Green, and Victoria D. Green
1996. NAGPRA Is Forever: Osteology and Repatriation of Skeletons. *Annual Review of Anthropology* 25:81-103.

Shermis, Stewart
1969. The Paleopathography of the Leavenworth Site (39CO9), Corson County, South Dakota. MA thesis, University of Kansas, Lawrence.

Shermis, Steward[sic.]
1982-1984. Domestic Violence in Two Skeletal Populations. *Ossa* 9/11:143-151

Smith, G. Hubert
1936. J.B. Trudeau's Remarks on the Indians of the Upper Missouri, 1794-95. *American Anthropologist* 38:565-568.

Stirling, Matthew W.
1924. Archeological Investigations in South Dakota. *Explorations and Field-work of the Smithsonian Institution in 1923*, pp. 66-71.

Steinbock, R. Ted
1976. *Paleopathological Diagnosis and Interpretation: Bone Diseases in Ancient Human Populations*. C.C. Thomas, Springfield, IL.

Strong, William Duncan
1940. From History to Prehistory in the Northern Great Plains. *Smithsonian Miscellaneous Collection* 100: 353-394.

Thomas, David Hurst
2000. *Skull Wars: Kennewick Man, Archaeology, and the Battle for Native American Identity*. Basic Books, New York.

Thompson, David (J.B. Tyrell, editor)
1916. *David Thompson's Narrative of His Explorations in Western America, 1784-1812*. The Champlain Society, Toronto.

Trudeau, Jean Baptiste
1914. Trudeau's Journal. *South Dakota Historical Collections* 7: 403-474.

Ubelaker, Douglas H.
1971. Appendix A. Dentition. IN W.M. Bass, D.R. Evans, and R.L. Jantz, The Leavenworth Site Cemetery: Archaeology and Physical Anthropology, *University of Kansas Publications in Anthropology*, no. 2, pp. 184-193.

2006. Populations Size, Contact to Nadir. IN D.H. Ubelaker (ed.) *Handbook of North American Indians: Environment, Origins and Population*, vol. 3, pp. 694-701. Smithsonian Institution Press, Washington, DC.

Vogel, F., and A.G. Motulsky
1997. *Human Genetics: Problems and Approaches.* Springer-Verlag, Berlin

Vogel, F., H.J. Pettenkofer, and W. Helmbold
1960. Uber die Populationsgenetik der ABO-Blutgruppen. *Actaicae Genet* 10: 267-294.

Walker, Ernest G.
1983. Evidence for Prehistoric Cardiovascular Disease of Syphilitic Origin on the Northern Plains. *American Journal of Physical Anthropology* 60: 499-503.

Wedel, Waldo R.
1955. Archeological Materials from the Vicinity of Mobridge, South Dakota. *Bureau of American Ethnology Bulletin* 157: 69-188. (Reprinted as Reprints in Anthropology, vol. 1, 1976, J & L Reprint Company, Lincoln, NE.)

Weiss, Elizabeth
2006. Research and NAGPRA. *American Committee for Preservation of Archaeological Collections (ACPAC) Newsletter*, September:1-2.

Weist, Katherine M.
1980 . Plains Indian Women: An Assessment. IN W.R. Wood and M. Liberty (eds.) *Anthropology on the Great Plains*, University of Nebraska Press, Lincoln. Pages 255– 271.

Willey, P.
1990. *Prehistoric Warfare on the Great Plains: Skeletal Analysis of the Crow Creek Massacre Victims.* Garland Publishing, New York.

Willey, P., and Thomas E. Emerson
1993. The Osteology and Archaeology of the Crow Creek Massacre. In "Prehistory and Human Ecology of the Western Prairies and Northern Plains," *Plains Anthropologist Memoir* 27, vol. 38, no. 145, pp. 227-269.

Willey, P., and Bob Mann
1986. The Skeleton of an Elderly Woman from the Crow Creek Site and Its Implications for Paleodemography. *Plains Anthropologist* 31(112):141-152.

Willey, P., and Mark Swegle
1980. A Sioux Child with Notched Teeth from South Dakota. *South Dakota Archaeology* 4:33-44.

Wood, W. Raymond
1980 . Plains Trade on Prehistoric and Protohistoric Intertribal Relations. IN W. R.Wood and M. Liberty (eds.) *Anthropology on the Great Plains*, University of Nebraska Press, Lincoln. Pages 98-109.

Index

Arikara:
    demography, 120-121, 129-131
    doctors, 92-95
    earthlodge, 72-73, 94
    economy, 73-74, 76
    elderly individuals, 131-132
    gardens, 73, 75
    generosity, 4, 20-21
    healing ceremony, 96
    illness from supernatural causes, 95
    incest, 46-47
    life expectancy, 130-132
    marriage pattern, 18, 42-44
    medicine, 95-107
    population, 70-72
    population decline, 121-122
    prostitutes, 30-33
    prostitution, 22-42
    remedies for diseases, 92-107
    seduction, 44-45, 46
    sex education, 42
    sex middlemen, 24-30
    sexual availability of women, 1-7,11-13, 151, 152, 153
    sexually transmitted diseases, 8, 55-58
    sexually transmitted diseases other than syphilis, 149
    spiritual power, 38-42
    trade, 2-5, 33-35, 38
    trade fair, 75-76

trade network, prehistoric, 74-78
villages (also see Leavenworth Site), 3, 25-29, 70-73
villages abandoned, 77-78
village location, 71
wealth, 4
women as source of syphilis, 91
women's beauty, 30, 32, 154
women's power, 28-29, 75
Arikara War, 25-28
    initiation, 2-27
    Leavenworth's siege, 27-28
Ashley, William Henry, 26-27
Bass, William M., 78, 79, 82
    estimation of Leavenworth Site population, 108-110
    skeletons excavated from Leavenworth Site, 78, 82
Beads, glass, 33-35
Bell, Benjamin, 52, 58
Biddle, Nicholas, 6
Brackenridge, Henry Marie, 104
    Arikara elderly, 131-132
    Arikara generosity, 21
    Arikara healing ceremony, 96
    Arikara polygamy, 43
    Arikara prostitution, 34
    Arikara sex middlemen, 29
    Arikara sexual availability, 16, 29, 30
    Arikara visit, 16
    Arikara women's beauty, 30-31
    background, 16
    prostitution clients, 36, 37
Bradbury, John:
    Arikara prostitution, 34-35
    Arikara treatment of illness, 101-102, 155
    Arikara sex middlemen, 29
    Arikara sexual availability, 15
    Arikara use of healing plants, 101-102, 104
    Arikara visit by, 13
    background, 13-15
    prostitution clients, 36
    sexually transmitted disease, 104
Brues, Alice, 127
Caddo:
    ABO Blood Type frequencies, 128-129
Cheyenne:
    visit Arikara villages, 4
Chlamydia:
    associated with Reiter's Syndrome, 60
    symptoms, 60
Clark, William:
    Arikara sexual availability, 1, 5-7

Arikara women's beauty, 30
    possibly fathered Nez Perce son, 48
Coneflower, purple, 105-106, 155
    Bradbury noted Arikara use of, 102, 104
    Bradbury's expedition members used to treat venereal disease, 104-105
    Lewis and Clark submit sample to Jefferson, 105
    other medicinal uses for, 105-106
Crow Creek Site:
    massacre and scalpings, 112
Daytime Smoker:
    possibly William Clark's son, 48
Denig, Edwin Thompson:
    Arikara incest, 46
    background, 44
    Indian seduction compared to war honor, 44-45, 46
    sexually transmitted disease, 57
Ft. Manuel Lisa, 17-18
Gass, Patrick:
    Arikara sexual availability, 1, 5
    Arikara women's beauty, 30
Gilmore, Melvin R., 100
Gonorrhea:
    causative microbe identified, 60, 89
    skeletal indicators, 64
    symptoms, 58, 60
    treatment, 54
Greggs, John and Pauline, 82, 83
Hayden, F.V.:
    background, 56
    syphilis among Arikara, 56-57
Holder, Preston, 78
Illness, 83
    epidemics, 76, 119
    smallpox, 121-123
Krause, Richard, 78
Leavenworth, Henry, 27-28, 77
Leavenworth Site, 78-82
    bone preservation, 116
    demography, 129-132, 135-136, 156, 157
    dental wear, 116-117
    excavations, 78, 152
    location, 71
    life expectancy, 109, 130-132
    years occupied, 108-109
Lewis, Meriwether:
    Arikara sexual availability, 1
Lewis and Clark Expedition, 1, 105-106, 120
    anticipation of sexually transmitted disease, 54
    sexually transmitted diseases mentioned, 48-49
Lewis and Clark Site (see Leavenworth Site)

Luttig, John C.:
    Arikara sex middlemen, 29
    Arikara sexual availability, 18, 29
    at Ft. Manuel Lisa, 17-18
    background, 16-17
    Sacagawea's death, 18
Mandan, 1, 3-4, 11, 48, 53
Medical thought, 89-90
    four humors, 51-52
NAGPRA (see Native American Graves Protection and Repatriation Act)
Native American Graves Protection and Repatriation Act (NAGPRA), 78, 145-148
    Kennewick man, 146-147
New Madrid Earthquake, 14-15
Omaha, 11, 100
Ordway, John:
    Arikara women's beauty, 30
Otoes, 1
Over, William, 78, 79, 82
Pawnee, 100
    ABO Blood Type frequencies, 128-129
Population decline:
    Arikara, 120-121
    Native Americans, 119-120
Rush, Benjamin, 90
Sacagawea:
    her death, 18
Saugrain, Antoine Francois, 90
Scalping, 17, 111
    bone alterations, 111-112
    tale of Scalped Man's Plight, 110-114, 157
Sex:
    vulva capture, 45
Shermis, Stewart, 82, 117-118
    infectious disease in Leavenworth Site skeletons, 83
Sioux (see Teton Dakota)
Skeletal age estimations:
    accuracy, 134-136
    standards, 134-135
Smallpox, 121-123
    eradication, 122-123
    forms, 122
    symptoms, 122
    virgin soil epidemic, 123
Stirling, Matthew W., 78, 79
Strong, William Duncan, 78, 79
Syphilis:
    and ABO Blood Types, 125-129, 157
    aortic aneuryism, 85
    causative microbe identified, 54, 60, 89
    changes in manifestations, 140-141, 158

congenital syphilis, early form, 63
congenital syphilis, late form, 63
congenital syphilis, symptoms, 63
congenital syphilis, skeletal indications, 68
distinguished from gonorrhea, 52, 89
epidemiology, 62-63
on the Plains, archaeology, 84-87
origin, 123-135
origin, Columbian Hypothesis, 124-125, 144-145
origin, PreColumbian Hypothesis, 125
rates, 133-134
skeletal indicators of, 64-68, 79, 86-87, 132, 136-137
studies of untreated individuals, 137
symptoms of, 57, 58, 61-62
treatment during 19th century, 53
treatment during 20th century, 54, 127
treatment and ABO Blood Types, 127-128
Tabeau, Pierre Antoine, 4-5
    Arikara generosity, 21
    Arikara illness, 95
    Arikara legermain, 95-96
    Arikara perspectives on whites, 38
    Arikara polygyny, 43
    Arikara sexual availability, 13
    Arikara sexually transmitted disease, 55
    Arikara sex middlemen, 24-25
    Arikara trade, 5, 34
    Arikara treatment of illness, 107
    Arikara women's ugliness, 32
    background, 12-13
    living with Arikara, 4-5
Teton Dakota, 1, 4, 6, 11, 100
Thompson, David:
    syphilis among Mandan, 56
Trade:
    Euroamerican, 76-77
    Prehistoric, 74-78
Traders (see Denig, Tabeau, Thompson, and Trudeau)
Travelers (see Brackenridge and Bradbury)
Trudeau, Jean Baptiste:
    among Arikara, 10-11, 35
    Arikara generosity, 20-21
    Arikara marriage, 42-43, 44
    Arikara population estimation, 120
    Arikara prostitution, 22, 24, 33-34
    Arikara sexual behavior, 11-12
    Arikara sex middlemen, 24
    Arikara treatment of venereal disease, 101
    background, 10-11
    prostitution clients, 36

school master, 11
sexually transmitted diseases, 55-56
Tuberculosis, 140-141
Ubelaker, Douglas H., 82
dental materials from Leavenworth Site skeletons, 82, 84
War of 1812, 17
York, 48
among the Arikara, 7
Arikara considered "medicine," 7, 41
claimed was originally a wild animal, 7
sexual activity with Arikara, 7, 41